Natural Proges

"*All of his recommendations are backed by the most informative and lucid explanation of the female hormone cycle that I've encountered. This book contains priceless information for women wrestling with the effects of menopause and hormone imbalance and for the doctors who treat them.*"

Julie Klotter in the
Townsend Letter for Doctors

Natural Progesterone

The multiple roles of a remarkable hormone

SECOND EDITION

John R. Lee, MD

Foreword by Dr Shirley Bond,
MB. BS. LRCP. MRCS. FFARCS.

JON CARPENTER

To order our books, please phone 01689 870437 or 01608 819117 and pay
by credit card, or send a cheque to the address below.
Postage is free within the UK.

Published in England by
Jon Carpenter Publishing, Alder House, Market Street, Charlbury, OX7 3PH
☎ 01608 811969

First edition published 1996, reprinted 1996, 1997

Second revised edition published 1999, reprinted 2002, 2003, 2010

ISBN 978 1 897766 54 5

Cover design by Sarah Tyzack

Printed in England by CPI Antony Rowe Ltd, Chippenham SN14 6LH

Contents

NOTE TO THE READER

This book describes the nature of progesterone hormone and its physiological functions. It is not intended to be a total replacement of standard medical care which has its place in the treatment of disease. This book is intended to educate physicians and lay people regarding progesterone and suggests the roles it may serve in application to health. **As with other hormones, any use of progesterone as a therapeutic modality should be undertaken only with consultation with one's physician.**

Neither the author nor the publisher can be held responsible for the use by an unqualified person of progesterone or any other hormone or drug described in this book.

Throughout this book, the abbreviation tsp refers to a teaspoon (5ml).

Foreword

MOST PRACTITIONERS, like myself, who are involved in the treatment of women with hormone imbalances, either at menopause or during their earlier reproductive life, are becoming increasingly aware that the pharmaceutically prepared hormones are not the complete answer.

This is especially noticeable with HRT which, over the years it has been available, has improved the quality of life for many menopausal women. However, while many women are fit and healthy on their HRT, many are not. They are affected by side effects, especially those due to the chemically altered progesterone included in HRT. Even women who have had hysterectomies and are prescribed oestrogen on its own suffer the effects of oestrogen dominance. Others are concerned about possible carcinogenic effects of HRT.

Many of these women stop HRT of their own accord, preferring to put up with the symptoms of the menopause itself.

Management of these women is difficult. Some of their symptoms can be helped by changes in their lifestyle, by diet and by vitamin supplementation.

When I came across the work of Dr John Lee and looked into it further, I felt that here might be an answer. In this book Dr Lee's theory and work is clearly and scientifically set out. It is interesting to note that the advantages of natural progesterone were well known prior to the introduction of the artificial progesterones in 1950. The introduction of a progestin which was easily absorbed by mouth and which could be supplied in a reliable, constant dosage seemed so easy. The contraceptive pill was introduced and HRT began to be used. Natural progesterone was forgotten by the medical profession. Now we have been reminded of it again by Dr Lee's work and — as I have found — by women who have heard about his work and want to use natural progesterone themselves.

Over the past three years I and several of my colleagues have treated menopausal women and women with PMS, irregular periods, miscarriages and osteoporosis. We are seeing some very interesting and promising responses to this treatment.

I would recommend that practitioners in this field read this book with an open mind, consider Dr Lee's work and research, and seriously consider including natural progesterone as part of their regime for dealing with the problems he discusses.

Dr Shirley Bond, MB. BS. LRCP. MRCS. FFARCS.

London, January 1996

Since I wrote the Foreword to the earlier edition of this book, nothing has happened to reduce my opinion as to the value of progesterone in the management of hormone imbalance. If anything I am appreciating its value more and more.

Fortunately, as a result of John Lee's lecture tours and Medical Letters, more and more women are aware of progesterone and realising its value. Consequently more and more doctors are becoming aware of progesterone and the fact that women want to use it. Sadly many of them are still not making themselves familiar with it and are sticking to traditional approaches. This must — and I am sure will — eventually change.

S.B., April 1999

Introduction

DISCOVERY, IT IS SAID, favours the prepared mind. Such preparedness may occur as a result of intentional study or may be accidental and/or serendipitous. In my case I credit serendipity. Some twenty-five years ago I was editor of our local medical society bulletin and responsible for a monthly editorial. Always casting about for topics of interest, I was facing a December editorial without any idea of a seasonally pertinent topic. During the week before the editorial due date, two intriguing articles crossed my desk. One was a *Harvard Alumni* journal article on the mystery of the Christmas mistletoe custom, i.e., a licence to kiss any lady standing under a sprig of mistletoe, a custom apparently originating with the Celts for reasons unknown. The other was a *JAMA* story of a doctor recently retired from a career at the NIH who had visited his boyhood hometown in Texas and, in conversation with a local gypsy lady renowned for her successful 'morning after' treatment for pregnancy prevention, discovered that her success involved the use of European mistletoe berries. The New World mistletoe lacked the essential ingredient for this effect. His subsequent analysis of the European mistletoe berry found an unexpected high concentration of progestational sterols, as well as other sterols and glycosides, including digitalis.

Here was a mystery to be solved. Did the progesterone in mistletoe berries have anything to do with the Celts' use of them and what connection could it have with the Christmas holiday? Consulting Frazer's *The Golden Bough* and other references I've long since forgotten, it is clear that our knowledge of the Celts comes primarily from the Roman historian, Pliny. European Celts, called Gauls by the Romans, revered oak-grown mistletoe (a saprophyte) for its multiple medicinal benefits (their name for it being 'All Heal'), as well as for its presumed sacred role, being sent by god as a sign of Life over Death. During the long frozen winters, the non-deciduous oaks, its mistletoe, and the evergreens are the only green and growing plants among the leafless trees of the vast snow-covered forests; and only mistletoe produces its berries in the dead of winter.

The physician-priest leaders of the Celts, the Druids, had for many centuries held a midwinter celebration timed to coincide with the winter solstice, starting on December 22-23 by our modern calender. The event, lasting a week, was meant to celebrate the promise that the sun would not disappear entirely and that the world would not die but would be rejuvenated by the return of the sun and the coming of Spring. Debts were paid in full, gifts exchanged, feasts were laid out, and a sacred concoction of hot mead laced with the revered berries, cut and collected in white cloth so as to not touch the ground, was plentifully supplied. We now know, of course, that progesterone stimulates libido and it is not difficult to imagine that whatever proscriptions there were against sexual licence were relaxed considerably under the influence of the warm alcohol and progesterone drink. We also know that menstrual shedding is the result of an abrupt fall in progesterone levels, which undoubtedly occurred when the week's carousing was over. Thus, any conception that occurred during the week of unrestricted sex would be lost with the induced menstrual flow, reinforcing the perception that festival sex without subsequent responsibility was merely another gift of the gods. When the midwinter week-long celebration was over, the leaders proclaimed the start of a new year and life among the Celts returned to normal.

The medicinal benefits of mistletoe were highly regarded throughout a number of different cultures of what is now Europe and elsewhere, even among the Aino of northern Japan. Concoctions of mistletoe were used to assist conception in humans and domesticated animals; to restore a zest of life; to cure epilepsy; to heal ulcers; and many other ailments. In a parallel to recent FDA pronouncements that deserves more attention, authorities of 'modern' times earlier this century declared that mistletoe had no medicinal value and was, in fact, dangerously poisonous. One might argue that the real message is that items of healing and health must be kept out the hands of ordinary folks and left strictly to the authorities and their professional guilds.

So it was that I wrote my Christmas editorial a quarter century ago on the subject of mistletoe, pointing out that the seasonal licence to kiss any woman standing under a twig of mistletoe was merely a pale reminder of the sexual licence enjoyed by the Celts during their winter solstice celebration, a gift of the natural progesterone, if not the gods, found in the mistletoe berry. As one might expect, I heard from a number of readers, some incensed that I had implied a non-Christian, perhaps pagan, relic appearing in the celebration of Christ's birth (but offering no other explanation for the custom); but others pointed out to me that this business of hormones in plants was not at all unusual in that over 5000 plants contain progesterone-like substances. The word phyto-hormone was not yet in vogue. A number of surprisingly tolerant responses came from theological school sources, also, asking for further references.

Some years later, in 1978 when I heard Dr. Ray Peat lecture on the subject of natural progesterone derived from wild yam root, the concept was not at all strange to me. I had been in practice long enough to realize that oestrogen along with calcium and vitamin D was not the complete answer for osteoporosis. Neither did I doubt that progesterone was absorbable transdermally. The fact that osteoporosis accelerated at the time of menopause strongly implicated the gonadal hormones. If oestrogen alone wasn't the answer, perhaps progesterone was also involved in keeping bones strong. Faced with menopausal osteoporotic patients unable to use oestrogen by reason of prior breast or uterine cancer or other contra-indications, it seemed entirely reasonable to me to offer them the option of using a progesterone skin cream moisturizer (Cielo) readily available over-the-counter.

In a further incidence of serendipity, Dr. Malcolm Powell had just recently opened a local facility offering relatively low cost dual photon absorptiometry (DPA), thus making accurate evaluation of bone mineral density a reality for those of us in clinical practice. To my considerable surprise, serial lumbar DPA tests showed actual increase, rather than mere delayed loss, in these patients. With that as encouragement, I broadened the scope of progesterone therapy to include patients already on oestrogen and found the same results. As if that were not enough, the patients reported improvement in other areas as well — increased alertness and energy, relief of breast fibrocysts and related mastodynia, recovery from mild hypothyroidism, decreased need of aspirin or anti-inflammatory drugs, normal blood pressure in those previously with mild hypertension, and, most un-expected of all, a return of normal libido. The icing on the cake was the fact of no hint of side effects.

As patient after patient showed the same pattern of benefits from transdermal natural progesterone, it did not take long to accumulate data to share with my colleagues. It was here, however, that another unexpected dimension of progesterone therapy arose: my colleagues applauded my presentations but, almost uniformly, chose not to apply the treatment to their patients. Their reasons were weak and self-serving, it seemed to me, invoking the fear of malpractice, their liability if perchance one of their patients developed a cancer, their concern about what colleagues might think, and the fact that no pharmaceutical company had undertaken to sponsor the treatment. Several, of course, called to inquire about details of my treatment plan since they wanted to use natural progesterone to treat their wives, mothers, or mothers-in-law. Over-riding all, however, was (1) their reliance on some official sanction before using natural progesterone instead of some synthetic progestin, and (2) their rather remarkable ignorance of hormone physiology. Given all the distractions of clinical practice, going 'by the book' requires much less effort (and is perceived a whole lot safer) than thinking for oneself, regardless of the potential benefit it might provide to the patient.

In the fifteen years since then, I have seen the consistent benefits and the safety of natural progesterone therapy. I have learned a great deal and obviously there is still more to learn. I have an urge to share what I have learned. You may call it mundane, but this is the simple reason I have written this book. I hope you enjoy reading it; you may even learn something from it and, in the process, reinforce the confidence and will power to act in the best tradition of being a physician scientist and a strong advocate for your patients.

John R. Lee, MD
Sebastopol, California
October 1993

1

A history of progesterone

ANIMAL HUSBANDRY AND HUMAN PROCREATION have fascinated man
since pre-Biblical times. Fertility symbols, rites, icons, and fetishes
abound in all cultures since the Stone Age. The regular occurrence of natural
breeding times, annually in some animals and monthly in women, was recognized several millennia before Christ. The early Greeks provided the word
'oestrus' (i.e., frenzy) and other cultures used their words for 'heat' to describe
the fruitful breeding times of female animals, including women. The causes
of these cyclic occurrences of oestrus were, of course, unknown.

Despite the deep attraction of the concept of fertility, the relative role of the
female was little understood throughout the Middle Ages. Woman was
considered the receptacle for the bearing (gestation, from the Latin *gestare*, to
carry or bear) of the germinating seed of man. It was not until the mid-1800s
that the female was understood to provide an equal share of the inherited
characteristics of her offspring, thus reviving a perplexing problem for the
Christian church, i.e., that of Jesus' insulation from Original Sin which had
previously been dealt with by a non literal translation of New Testament texts
removing Mary's husband, Joseph, from Jesus' parentage. In 1854, the bull
of Pius IX proclaimed the dogma of the Immaculate Conception by which
Mary is said to have been conceived and born without Original Sin. Thus
does science influence ecclesiastic thought.

In 1866, Gregor Mendel, an obscure Austrian monk, published his paper on
hybridization of peas describing the equal importance of male and female
factors to inherited characteristics of succeeding plant generations. Despite the
impetus stemming from the independent but simultaneous publications in
1858 by C. R. Darwin and A. R. Wallace, as well as Darwin's superb and very
successful *Origin of Species* (1859), all dealing with inherited factors of selection
as the modus operandi for evolution, Mendel's work was essentially ignored
at the time. However, these genetic principles were rediscovered a generation
later in 1900 by three scientists, Hugo de Vries, C. G. Correns, and Erich
Tschermak-Seysenegg, each working independently in different countries.

Not only did the science of genetics make a quantum leap during these years but so also did the science of the biochemistry of reproduction. In 1900, the ovaries' role in the hormonal control of the female reproductive system was established by Knauer. That same year, Halban showed that, if ovaries were implanted in immature animals, normal sexual development and function were assured. A simple, quantitative bioassay, based on vaginal smears in rats, for measuring ovarian extracts was developed by Allen and Doisy in 1923. In 1925, Frank et al reported the detection of an active sex principle in the blood of sows in oestrus. More importantly, in 1926, Lowe and Lange discovered a female sex hormone in the urine of menstruating women and observed that the concentration of the hormone varied with the phase of the menstrual cycle. In 1928, even greater amounts of this oestrus hormone, now called oestrogen, was found by Zondek in the urine of pregnant women, a finding which soon led to the isolation of the active substance in crystalline form (Butenandt, 1929; Doisy et al, 1929, 1930).[1]

During these fertile (no pun intended) years, early investigators postulated that the ovary produced two hormonal substances. In particular, Beard, in 1897, suggested that the small yellowish bodies (the corpora lutea) found on the ovary surface in pregnant females must serve a necessary function during pregnancy. This theory was supported by Fraenkel in 1903 when he showed that destruction of the corpora lutea in pregnant rabbits caused abortion. Finally, Corner and Allen, in 1929, firmly established the existence of the corpus luteum hormone which was necessary for the successful promotion of gestation (called progesterone) by showing that abortion following extirpation of the corpora lutea could be prevented by injection of luteal extracts. Shortly thereafter, they isolated the pure hormone from the corpora lutea of sows.[1] For several years, research was hampered by the small amount of progesterone that could be obtained in this manner. However, by the late 1930s, the placenta was found to synthesize progesterone in prodigious amounts (300-400 mg/day during the third trimester) in humans[2] and this led to the harvesting of placentas after childbirth and quick-freezing them for extraction of progesterone in quantities sufficient for experimental work and clinical application. A new era in medicine had dawned.

Progesterone was found to be a fat soluble compound which, when given orally, was relatively ineffective due to extensive and rapid first-pass metabolism in the liver. When dissolved in vegetable oil and given by injection, it is rapidly absorbed and thoroughly effective. However, when injected intramuscularly, progesterone in amounts over 100 mg is locally irritating (painful), somewhat limiting its use. Physicians attuned to the intricacies of hormone balance, however, found progesterone to be remarkably effective in patients with what is now called PMS, in treating ovarian cysts, and preventing threatened abortion. Aqueous suspensions were found to be even more painful and were seldom used. Progesterone is well absorbed when given transrectally or transvaginally, however. These methods of giving progesterone are still commonly used in Europe and England. Katherine Dalton of London has become world famous for treating premenstrual syndrome with transrectal progesterone.

Early in the 1950s, active oestrogen and progesterone-like sterol analogues were found in many plant varieties, now numbering in the 1000's. In particular, the sterol, diosgenin, is abundant in wild yams (Dioscorea). From it, natural progesterone is derived as a major, relatively inexpensive pharmaceutical product.

Due to the profit-making advantage of patentable compounds, pharmaceutical funding for progesterone research veered in the direction of patentable progesterone analogues synthesized from the yam-derived natural progesterone, leading to the introduction of new classes of progestational agents with prolonged activity and enhanced oral effectiveness. Such agents are referred to as progestins, progestogens, and gestagens, all meaning the same thing: any synthetically derived compound with the ability to sustain the human secretory endometrium. Unfortunately, progestins do not provide the full spectrum of natural progesterone's biological activity nor are they as safe. Despite their long list of safety concerns (see Chapter 3), progestins have become popular because of their effectiveness in birth control and protection against the oestrogen-induced risk of endometrial cancer. Research of natural progesterone has, in the past two decades, been essentially non-existent. Thus does industrial profit influence the path of science.

In my case, I had graduated from the University of Minnesota Medical School, completed a rotating internship (now called residency) at Minneapolis General Hospital, spent a good portion of a year in practice with a wizard physician in Faribault, Minnesota, and completed two interesting years in the Pacific area as a medical officer in the US. Navy and, in 1959, opened my own general practice of medicine in Mill Valley, California. I felt confident and well trained. I had diagnosed two cases of Cushing's disease that had gone undetected in others' offices, one pheochromocytoma, a parasaggital meningioma, a cerebral aneurysm in a lady referred to me as an hysteric (all in the days before CT scans and MRIs), a case of filariasis (in a daughter of a family recently returned from Africa), one case of hepatic amoebic histolytica, delivered babies, and managed a case of eclampsia. I was good at explaining the workings of birth control pills and had become an editor of our medical society's monthly journal. But there were also those women who came to me with premenstrual bloating, water retention, and emotional problems who told me that their previous doctor (usually an older, highly intelligent one back East) had treated them successfully with 'progesterone shots'. My treatments of diuretics, birth control hormones, or mild tranquillizers were usually unsuccessful and our local pharmacies no longer carried injectable progesterone. The era of natural progesterone had been short-lived and had come and gone before my time, swamped by the flood of synthetic hormones.

Recently, however, the advantage of natural progesterone has again become evident and its use in clinical situations is growing due to an interesting synchronicity of several factors. Osteoporosis is the major disabling disease of women in the US and its treatment by oestrogen is less than satisfactory.[3-7] Also, oestrogen imposes a risk of endometrial cancer which is largely preventable by progesterone and its analogues.[8] Third, accurate evaluation of bone mineral density is no longer in the domain of researchers but is attainable in everyday office practice. And last but not least, natural progesterone is efficiently absorbed transdermally, a fact that enhances patients' acceptance of its use and greatly reduces the cost of therapy. In 1980, when my 40-year old housewives had become 60-year olds with osteoporosis and I learned of transdermal natural progesterone (being sold as a skin moisturizer), I started adding it to my therapeutic regimen for osteoporosis, at first only to those for whom oestrogen was contraindicated. To my surprise, serial bone mineral density tests showed a significant rise without a hint of side effects. With this obvious success, my use of natural progesterone spread to osteoporosis patients who were not doing all that well on oestrogen alone. Again, it proved successful. (See Chapter 11.)

Eventually I wrote a paper[9] describing the success of natural progesterone and, bit by bit, became an advisor for others wishing to use the real progesterone. With more experience, it became clear that natural progesterone contributed to good health in women for a variety of problems and the word gradually spread. Physicians who once left the intricacies of hormone balance to gynaecologist and endocrinologist consultants returned to their textbooks to re-learn the lessons they had so long ignored. They discovered that progesterone is the major precursor of cortisone synthesis by the adrenal cortex; that oestrogen unopposed by progesterone is a factor in many symptom-complexes presenting in their offices daily, especially PMS; that fibrocystic breasts return to normal when adequate progesterone is supplied; that bones do become stronger when progesterone is added to the therapeutic program; that progesterone protects against breast cancer: that progesterone facilitates thyroid hormone activity and protects against salt and water retention, and, thus, hypertension; that transdermal progesterone is wonderful for skin hydration; and that their patients just plain feel better when progesterone deficiency is corrected.

The full history of progesterone is yet to be written. The scientific progress in the discovery and understanding of this remarkable hormone within just this century is amazing, of course, but even more is yet to come. The era of natural progesterone is not over; it is merely emerging from the flood of progestins. The chapters that follow will stir your interest, to say the least.

2

What is progesterone?

PROGESTERONE IS ONE of two main hormones, the other being oestrogen, made by ovaries of menstruating women. More specifically, it is the hormone made by the corpus luteum starting just prior to ovulation and increasing rapidly after ovulation to become the major female gonadal hormone during the latter two weeks of the menstrual cycle. It is necessary for the survival of the fertilized ovum, the resulting embryo, and the foetus throughout gestation when the synthesis of progesterone is taken over by the placenta. Progesterone is also made in smaller amounts by the adrenal glands in both sexes and by the testes in males, being an important step in the biosynthesis of adrenal cortical hormones. Its three major functions are (1) the survival and development of the conceptus, (2) a broad range of intrinsic biologic properties, and (3) its role as precursor of other steroid hormones.

The synthesis of progesterone originates in the ovary as a product of cholesterol which is, itself, synthesized from acetate (small, 2-carbon fragments obtained from catabolism of sugar and fatty acids). From progesterone are derived not only the other sex hormones but also the corticosteroids.

The pivotal position of progesterone in the biosynthetic pathway is clear. It participates in the ultimate formation of the corticosteroids and all the other sex hormones, i.e., the oestrogens and testosterone. In addition, it has vital intrinsic properties of its own and is the hormone most essential to the survival of the fertilized egg and the resulting conceptus, as we shall see.

In ovulating females, progesterone is chiefly produced by the ovary (i.e., the corpus luteum) with smaller amounts made in the adrenal cortex in both sexes, and in the testes of males. Within the cytoplasm of cells are minute organelles, the mitochondria, which convert cholesterol to pregnenolone which, on being transferred to the cytoplasm, is converted to progesterone or DHEA, depending on cell type and body needs. With the development of the corpus luteum and ovulation (see Chapter 8), the ovarian production of progesterone rapidly rises from 2-3 mg per day to an average of 22 mg per day, peak production being as high as 30 mg per day, a week or so after ovulation.

After ten or twelve days, if fertilization does not occur, ovarian production of progesterone falls dramatically. It is this sudden decline in progesterone levels that triggers the shedding of the secretory endometrium (the menses) leading to a renewal of the entire menstrual cycle. During pregnancy, production of progesterone is taken over by the placenta which secretes an ever-increasing supply, reaching 300-400 mg per day during the third trimester.

Progesterone, as it is secreted into the blood stream, is bound within a water-soluble protein (termed cortisol binding globulin [CBG], being the same globulin used by cortisol for passage through the plasma). Only a small portion of progesterone (2-10%) circulates unbound through the plasma. The molecular framework of progesterone, having been derived from cholesterol, is very similar to the cholesterol molecule and, like cholesterol, is fat soluble. As such, it would not be soluble in the watery plasma were it not for the CBG protein carrier.

Cholesterol molecules are major components of cell membranes each of which, from the perspective of a molecule that small, is rather like a webbed bag holding the cell together but with sufficient spaces between molecules for the passage of oxygen, carbon dioxide, specific minerals and other similarly minute substances. In close proximity to a cell, progesterone is freed from the CBG and floats easily through cell membranes into the cell cytoplasm where, if it encounters and binds to an accessible receptor, forms an activated complex which migrates into the cell nucleus for binding with an accessible DNA segment (genome) resulting in the formation of specific RNA by which the cellular effects of progesterone are brought into being. If the progesterone floats into a cell lacking an appropriate progesterone receptor, it will simply float on through and out the cell again. That is the nature of all hormone function.

Eventually, progesterone molecules are carried by the blood through the liver where they are inactivated (metabolized) and disposed of via the bile and urine. The inactivation process involves the addition of hydrogen at various double bond sites of its molecular structure (a process called hydrogenation, or reduction) leading to the formation of three closely related groups of compounds; pregnanediones, pregnanalones, and pregnanediols. These inactive metabolites are then conjugated with glucuronic acid and excreted as water-soluble glucuronides primarily in bile but also in the urine. Urinary pregnanediol is used as an index of endogenous production levels of progesterone.

The role of progesterone in human metabolism and physiologic functions will be summarized here. More detailed descriptions will be given in various of the following chapters as indicated in the table of contents.

I. Procreation

As indicated in Chapter 1, progesterone was found to be the hormone that makes possible the survival of the fertilized egg. It is produced by the corpus luteum of the matured ovarian follicle from which the ovum emerges. Progesterone is given its name for its function in promoting gestation. It maintains the secretory endometrium which the fertilized ovum will invade and from which the germinating egg (blastoderm) and the resultant embryo will gain sustenance during its trophoblastic stage. As might be expected, the surge of progesterone at the time of ovulation is the source of libido, the urge to procreate, by which is meant the sexual drive to bring ovum and sperm together.

Progesterone is necessary to prevent the premature shedding of the supportive secretory endometrium. Any drop in progesterone level or blockade of its receptor sites at this time will result in the loss of the embryo (abortion). This, in fact, is the action of the anti-progesterone compound, RU-486. As the placenta develops, it assumes and progressively increases the production of progesterone for the duration of the gestation period, i.e. until birth of the baby. During the third trimester, progesterone is produced at the rate of >300 mg/day, an astounding level for hormone production which, for other hormones, is usually measured in micrograms per day. In some countries, placentas are harvested after delivery of the baby and used for extraction of their progesterone content.

Progesterone (unlike oestrogen and testosterone) is devoid of secondary sex characteristics. Thus, its effects in promoting the development of the foetus are independent of the baby's gender. The foetus is allowed to develop according to its own DNA code and not be affected by the hormones of the mother.

II. Intrinsic biologic properties

Progesterone has many beneficial actions throughout the body. The list below provides an indication of its diversity and importance. Since progesterone protects against the undesirable side effects of unopposed oestrogen, whether occurring endogenously before menopause or as a consequence of oestrogen supplementation, these effects will be included in the list. Oestrogen, it should be recalled, allows influx of water and sodium into cells, thus affecting

Figure 1. Biosynthetic pathway of sex and adrenal hormones

aldosterone production leading to water retention and hypertension. Oestrogen causes intra-cellular hypoxia, opposes the action of thyroid, promotes histamine release, promotes blood clotting thus increasing the risk of stroke and embolism, thickens bile and promotes gall bladder disease, and causes copper retention and zinc loss. Oestrogen, unopposed by progesterone, decreases libido, increases the likelihood of breast fibrocysts, uterine fibroids, uterine (endometrial) cancer and breast cancer. All of these undesirable effects of oestrogen are countered by progesterone. Restoring proper progesterone levels is what is known as restoring hormone *balance.*

Functions of progesterone
- precursor of other sex hormones, i.e., oestrogen and testosterone
- maintains secretory endometrium
- protects against breast fibrocysts
- is a natural diuretic
- helps use fat for energy
- is a natural antidepressant
- helps thyroid hormone action
- normalizes blood clotting
- restores libido
- helps normalize blood sugar levels
- normalizes zinc and copper levels
- restores proper cell oxygen levels
- protects against endometrial cancer
- helps protect against breast cancer
- stimulates osteoblast-mediated bone building
- necessary for survival of embryo and foetus throughout gestation
- precursor of cortisone synthesis by adrenal cortex

Each of these will be discussed more thoroughly in the chapters to follow.

Before discussing the third important function of progesterone, its role in steroid synthesis, it may be helpful to review the biosynthesis of cholesterol and of pregnenolone, also. Cholesterol can be synthesized by cells throughout the body, particularly in the liver, from acetate, a 2-carbon fragment derived from starches and/or fat. In broad outline, the first stage is the formation of aceto-acetyl-sulphated coenzyme A. The final steps are the oxidation and cyclization of squalene.

The biosynthesis of steroid hormones begins with the conversion of cholesterol to pregnenolone. Cholesterol is first taken up into the mitochon-

dria where it is sequentially hydroxylated at C-20 and C-22 followed by cleavage of the bond between these two sites to form pregnenolone. The overall controllers of steroid biosynthesis are the three pituitary hormones, ACTH, LH and FSH.

III. Steroid precursor function

The steroid precursor function of progesterone deserves some special attention. Hormone synthesis is a dynamic fluctuating system, responding to changing body conditions and needs. Hormones are the messengers of control of a vast, interrelated, ever-changing network of organ-system commands. As such, they must be continually created for moment-to-moment situational needs; and, likewise, must be metabolized and removed from the system when no longer needed in order for their presence to rise and fall as their need changes. Metabolism of steroid hormones is an ongoing process within the liver. Progesterone, in addition to its own intrinsic hormonal effects, is a main player in the biosynthesis of all these hormones. Various cells in key organs throughout the body use progesterone to create the other specific hormones as needed, specifically, the adrenal corticosteroids, oestrogen, and testosterone.

This aspect of progesterone distinguishes it from most other hormones which are at a metabolic end-point; i.e., unable to be used in further metabolic function except to be metabolized for excretion. More specifically, the various synthetic analogues of progesterone now being promoted heavily have undergone molecular alterations at unusual positions that inhibit further metabolism (and thus can not be 'turned off' to prevent excessive or improperly prolonged activity). The not-found-in-Nature analogues produced pharmaceutically are heavily marketed because the analogues are patentable and therefore more profitable. Unfortunately, the molecular alterations carry a heavy burden of potential undesirable side effects. This, however, does not seem to deter the marketing of them. Physicians who are the targets of heavy pharmaceutical advertising (and unaware that natural progesterone is available) tend to accede to marketing pressure. Just as protein intake (i.e., an adequate supply of the essential amino acids) is necessary for the production of peptide hormones and enzymes, so is natural progesterone needed for the appropriate and balanced supply of all the steroid hormones. To overcome present marketing practices and restore natural progesterone to its proper place in the practice of medicine will apparently require re-education of its diverse and important role in health by patients and doctors alike.

In summary, this valuable hormone maintains secretory endometrium, is essential for survival and development of the conceptus, protects against oestrogen side effects, is an important precursor in the biosynthetic pathway for other sex hormones and the adrenal corticosteroids, and its levels of activity in response to body needs are controlled by the balance between its production from cholesterol and its metabolism and excretion by the liver. See Figure 1.

As can be seen, progesterone is a key player, being the precursor of adrenal steroids as well as a precursor of testosterone and oestrogens. At first glance, most readers are impressed by what seems to be a remarkable similarity in molecular 'chassis', if you will, of all these compounds. They are all composed of four rings similar to the lettered rings in the cholesterol configuration. Progesterone and testosterone, differ only by the molecular fragment attached at C-17 (the tip of the D ring). In particular, the A ring of each contains a double bonded oxygen at C-3 and a double bond between C-4 and C-5. These changes in the A ring result in potent stereochemical and electromagnetic differences from cholesterol and may account for a commonality of receptor sites among progesterone, testosterone, and corticosterone, such as is found in osteoblast bone cells.

Interestingly, though all three of these hormones compete for the same receptors within osteoblasts, the action they induce is strikingly different. Both progesterone and testosterone stimulate new bone formation by osteoblasts; corticosteroids' action, however, is to 'turn off' osteoblast-mediated new bone formation. Just as specific keys operate specific locks, the function of any given hormone is dependent upon its specific molecular configuration. Minute differences in molecular structure convey vastly different biological effects.

The A ring of oestrogens, on the other hand, has become aromatized by three sets of double bonds (as in benzene) and hydroxylated at C-3, and is now called phenolated due to its similarity to phenol. This major difference in the A ring of oestrogens connotes major differences in receptor sites and metabolic effects when compared, for instance, to progesterone and testosterone, both of which are anti-oestrogenic in action.

Let us now take a look at the difference between progesterone and the progestins.

3

What are progestins?

PROGESTINS ARE OFTEN DEFINED as any compound able to sustain the human secretory endometrium. Thus, many writers will include natural progesterone in the general class of progestins. Progesterone, however, is the only such hormone made by the body and has many important functions which are not provided by synthetic progestins. The problem of recognizing the uniqueness of progesterone is made worse by the common semantic error of reversing the concept of hormone class; i.e., many writers fall into the pattern of referring to progestin as being in the general class of progesterones, apparently not realizing that there is but one progesterone, the specific molecule made by the ovary. The general confusion is made even worse by the European writers who refer to progestins as gestagens; and others use the word, progestogens. To maintain clarity of thought, I would choose to define progestins as any compound, other than natural progesterone, able to sustain human secretory endometrium.

This chapter, therefore, will explain why the prevailing assumption is unwarranted that synthetic progestins are equivalent to natural progesterone. One rather clear example is the fact that progesterone is *necessary* for the survival and development of the embryo and throughout gestation whereas Provera, the most commonly prescribed progestin, carries the warning that its use in early pregnancy may *increase* the risk of early abortion or congenital deformities of the foetus. This is but one of the many differences between progesterone and the seven most commonly prescribed synthetic progestins, two of which (medroxyprogesterone acetate and megestrol acetate) are synthesized from the 21-carbon nucleus of progesterone, and the other five (norgestrel, norethindrone acetate, norethynodrel, lynestrenol and norethisterone (norethindrone)) from the 19-carbon nucleus of nortestosterone.

The reader may note that the pharmaceutical progestins do not appear in the biosynthetic pathway picture in Figure 1. The fact is, they are not found in any living forms. They are synthetically derived, most commonly from progesterone itself or from testosterone, and can be synthesized *de novo* but this is more

Potential side effects of medroxyprogesterone acetate (Provera)

Warnings:

Increased risk of birth defects such as heart and limb defects if taken during the first four months of pregnancy.

Beagle dogs given this drug developed malignant mammary nodules.

Discontinue this drug if there is sudden or partial loss of vision.

This drug passes into breast milk, consequences unknown.

May contribute to thrombophlebitis, pulmonary embolism, and cerebral thrombosis.

Contraindications:

Thrombophlebitis, thromboembolic disorders, cerebral apoplexy; liver dysfunction or disease; known or suspected malignancy of breast or genital organs, undiagnosed vaginal bleeding; missed abortion; or known sensitivity.

Precautions:

May cause fluid retention, epilepsy, migraine, asthma, cardiac or renal dysfunction.

May cause breakthrough bleeding or menstrual irregularities.

May cause or contribute to depression.

The effect of prolonged use of this drug on pituitary, ovarian, adrenal, hepatic, or uterine function is unknown.

May decrease glucose tolerance; diabetic patients must be carefully monitored.

May increase the thrombotic disorders associated with oestrogens.

Adverse Reactions:

May cause breast tenderness and galactorrhoea.

May cause sensitivity reactions such as urticaria, pruritus, oedema, or rash.

May cause acne, alopecia and hirsutism.

Oedema, weight changes (increase or decrease).

Cervical erosions and changes in cervical secretions.

Cholestatic jaundice

Mental depression, pyrexia, nausea, insomnia or somnolence.

Anaphylactoid reactions and anaphylaxis (severe acute allergic reactions).

Thrombophlebitis and pulmonary embolism.

Breakthrough bleeding, spotting, amenorrhoea, or changes in menses.

When taken with oestrogens, the following have been observed:

Rise in blood pressure, headache, dizziness, nervousness, fatigue

Changes in libido, hirsutism and loss of scalp hair, decrease in T-3 uptake values.

Premenstrual-like syndrome, changes in appetite.

Cystitis-like syndrome.

Erythema multiforme, erythema nodosum, haemorrhagic eruption, itching.

expensive and therefore uncommon. Note that the differences from progesterone are relatively minor but these differences are nevertheless significant. Each of these molecules represents a metabolic end-point. The atoms introduced at unusual positions will inhibit their metabolism and prolong their activity as well as induce actions which are not consistent with that of natural progesterone. (Furthermore, being foreign to all living things, they are patentable and thereby potentially more profitable.)

A distinction is sometimes made between C-21 and C-19 progestins. C-21 agents (having a 21-carbon nucleus of progesterone) have little or no effect on lipids whereas C-19 agents (having a 19-carbon nucleus of nortestosterone) are thought to diminish the presumed beneficial effect of oestrogen on lipids. Some writers, in their semantic confusion between progestins and progesterone, have mistakenly written that *progesterone* may have an adverse effect on serum lipids when, in fact, it does not.[1] In general, progesterone has a beneficial effect of improving serum lipid profiles.[2]

Progestins of both the C-21 and C-19 variety have been found to be well absorbed when applied transdermally,[3,4] a capacity shared by natural progesterone, oestrogen, and testosterone. All are relatively small, fat-soluble compounds that pass through the dermis (skin) easily and efficiently. It should be recalled that oral administration results in absorption and transportation to the liver where storage in fat occurs and eventual excretion via bile. The natural hormones are more quickly metabolized and excreted than the synthetic versions.

It should be clear that the basic body of the synthetic hormones (especially the A ring) remains identical to progesterone or nortestosterone and thus these compounds will likely bind with the same receptor sites as the natural hormones. However, the alterations (e.g., acetate or ethinyl groups) linked to the C-17 site will convey a different 'message' to the target cell. This undoubtedly explains the alarming array of listed warnings, contraindications, precautions, and adverse reactions, all of which are uncharacteristic of progesterone itself. Further, each progestin agent differs the other in terms of potency, progesterone effects, anti-progesterone effects, oestrogen effects, anti-oestrogen effects, androgenic (masculinizing) effects and many others. It is likely, therefore, that they differ also from progesterone in its bone-building effect.

Many physicians mistakenly believe that a progestin such as Provera (medroxyprogesterone acetate) is, somehow, the same as progesterone and thus believe that progesterone shares Provera's side effects when, in fact, progesterone has no known side effects. When Hargrove et al (1989) compared oral progesterone with medroxyprogesterone acetate in combined hormonal therapy with oestrogen for menopausal women, they found superior symptomatic improvement, an improved lipid profile, amenorrhoea without endometrial proliferation or hyperplasia, and no side effects in the group given progesterone.[2] All ten of the oestradiol/progesterone group wished to continue their hormone regimen, whereas two of the five women using conjugated oestrogen and medroxyprogesterone acetate requested discontinuation of their hormonal therapy due to side effects.

To appreciate the scope of progestin side effects, it is instructive to review the Physicians Desk Reference (PDR) pages for medroxyprogesterone acetate. An abbreviated list from the 1993 PDR is shown on page 18.

A side effect of both oestrogen and the progestins not sufficiently recognized by physicians is their effect on hypertension. Crane, for example, has extensively examined the effect of oestrogens, progestins, and progesterone on intracellular sodium influx and on the renin-aldosterone system.[5,6] Under conditions of health, a cell's membrane will selectively transfer potassium and magnesium into the cell while protecting against the influx of sodium. It has been known at least since 1972 that oestrogen promotes salt and water retention, thus increasing the risk of hypertension, and that oral contraceptives (combined oestrogen and progestin) led to elevated plasma renin activity. Renin is a hormone made by the kidney which promotes the conversion of angiotensinogen to anigiotensin I which, on being hydrolyzed to the active form, angiotensin II, stimulates the adrenal to produce the hormone aldosterone, a mineralcorticoid. Aldosterone, in turn, stimulates sodium retention by its resorption in the distal and collecting tubules of the kidney and promotes the potassium loss. This is the renin-aldosterone system which increases arterial pressure. Under conditions of severe salt restriction, this system is activated by the body to prevent an undesirable fall of arterial pressure.

Natural progesterone, on the other hand, is known to cause sodium diuresis with a secondary increase in aldosterone excretion rate, i.e. an 'anti-aldosterone' effect protecting against hypertension. Contemporary medicine assumes progestins are equivalent to natural progesterone. Crane and others[7,8] found that all oestrogens tested increased plasma renin substrate and sodium and water retention with variable effects on plasma renin activity; and all increased aldosterone excretion rate. The four progestins tested varied considerably in their action with norethindrone having oestrogenic effects and two others (medroxyprogesterone acetate and ethynodiol acetate), suppressing aldosterone production, interpreted as a mineralcorticoid effect of these steroids. None of the progestins were equivalent to natural progesterone in their renin-aldosterone effects.

When tested for sodium retention, the administration of progesterone induced sodium excretion whereas all four progestins increased sodium retention. Thus, when combined with oestrogens as in oral contraceptives, the progestins increase the risk of hypertension whereas progesterone protects against it. This is but another example of the significant differences between progesterone and the progestins.

Given all that is known about the great difference of actions and of safety between progesterone and the synthetic progestins, why is it that they have come to dominate in the role of progesterone supplementation? The answer lies in their use in contraceptive pills. The twin impediments to unrestricted sexual activity, especially by young, unattached adults, were the twin fears of unwanted pregnancy and venereal disease. In industrialized western culture, the development of the automobile effectively removed the young from their usual adult chaperones. The advent of penicillin and the apparent easy cures of gonorrhoea and syphilis removed the perceived threat of venereal disease. All that was needed for the explosion of the sexual freedom movement was a convenient, effective (and private) contraceptive. Thus was the stage set for progestational drugs.

When progesterone was obtainable (by commercial synthesis from plant fats and oils) in sufficient amounts for aggressive research by private biochemical industries, it did not take long for the development of oral, highly effective, synthetic progestins. It should be recalled that monthly ovarian follicle maturation proceeds in both ovaries until ovulation occurs in one of them, creating the corpus luteum which is responsible for a great surge of progesterone production. This surge of progesterone, as one of its effects, stops ovulation in the other ovary. (Which is why fraternal twins are born only once for every 300 pregnancies.) If sufficient progesterone is provided prior to ovulation, neither ovary produces an egg. This inhibition of ovulation is the original mechanism of action of progestin contraception. Accumulated experience and the occurrence of obvious side effects led to trials with progressively smaller doses. It was found that effective contraception with fewer obvious side effects could be obtained with such small doses as 0.5 mg of norethindrone or 0.3 mg of norgestrol, for example. These small doses are sufficient to suppress gonadotropins so that the gonadal (ovarian) hormone production is suppressed, resulting in an inhospitable (to fertilized ova) endometrium and thicker cervical mucus (which makes sperm passage more difficult) as well as inhibiting ovulation.

The advantage of progestins was (1) ease of delivery system [oral tablets], (2) consistent potency [guaranteed contraception], (3) longer duration of action [inability of the body to metabolize them], and (4) a patentable [i.e. profitable] product. Recall that these were the days when progesterone supplementation required expensive, painful injections or rectal or vaginal suppositories. The long lists of undesirable and potentially serious side effects from progestins are dutifully printed in the PDR and in product information sheets, usually in type so small that only the most curious and with good eyesight would read them. No one really wanted to know of them because of what was being offered: sex without fear of pregnancy.

Then came the problem with supplemental oestrogen. During the 1970s, it became obvious that postmenopausal women taking unopposed oestrogen for hot flushes, prevention of osteoporosis, or whatever, were at increased risk of endometrial cancer.[9,10] This rarely, if ever, occurred during one's fertile years when normal levels of endogenous oestrogen and progesterone were present. Testing postmenopausal women with combined hormone therapy (using both oestrogen and a progestin) found that oestrogen-induced endometrial cancer could be largely prevented. In the mid-70s, a Mayo Clinic consensus conference concluded that oestrogen should *never* be given to any woman with an intact uterus without also giving progesterone or a progestin to protect them from endometrial carcinoma. The effect of this was to expand the market for progestins to include all women, whether menstruating or postmenopausal! The financial implications of this are difficult to exaggerate.

A question not often discussed is: if oestrogen unopposed by progesterone is unwise when given after menopause, why isn't it equally unwise to allow endogenous oestrogen to be unopposed in the pre- or perimenopausal period?

A further complication, however, is the 1989 report by Bergkvist et al who rather convincingly showed that supplemental oestrogen (at least oestradiol) when combined with a progestin 'seems to be associated with a slightly *increased* risk of breast cancer, which is not prevented and may even be *increased* by the addition of the progestins.'[11] (Emphasis added.) This has not slowed the progestin bandwagon. (Natural progesterone, as we shall see in Chapter 12, helps prevent breast cancer.)

Our present situation regarding progestins is not difficult to understand. Chemically-altered progesterone is touted as the expedient prevention of pregnancy and endometrial cancer, and the treatment of an ever-widening pool of female complaints. Well-financed industry-supported academics view menopause, hot flushes, emotional changes, and osteoporosis as merely the result of hormone deficiency diseases easily managed with pharmaceutical chemicals for which they, the health scientists, are the master providers. Women, of course, do not take kindly to the notion that their lives are reduced to mere disorders or diseases. Upset they should be. Further, they should also be upset that the hormone 'balancing' being done to them uses synthetic and abnormal versions of the real goods when the natural hormones are available, safer, and more appropriate to their bodies.

Are progestins the wave of the future? One should hope not. Our goal should be that, when hormone therapy is indicated, the hormones should be the natural ones. It can be taken as a rule that, among steroids, any change in the molecular configuration will alter the steroid's effects. It should be clear that, given no change in ecologic constraints, evolutionary imperatives produce compounds that serve us best. Thus, natural progesterone is far more likely to be the compound of choice in restoring appropriate hormone levels, should such be indicated.

4

The dance of the steroids

U NDERSTANDING STEROIDS REQUIRES a vision into the unseen. Humans have the power to create reality beyond their normal experience. Actually we do it all the time in music, books, childhood stories, fantasy, dreams, and, yes, especially in science. Science is really the art of 'seeing' forces and elements invisible to the normal senses. No scientist has ever seen an atom, yet he conjures an image to understand them. He knows that the essential nature of all matter is really a form of electromagnetic force and that the apparent solidity of matter is a perception that devolves from the limitations of our sensory equipment. Einstein changed man's concept of reality by his equation. $E = MC^2$, equating mass with energy, in which E is energy, M is mass, and C is the velocity of light. We know that atoms can join together to create molecules; and the nature of their bonding involves a mystery of sharing electrons. But, by the rules we derive from Nature's hidden forces, we learn to understand, to use, and even to create molecules. In this chapter I will try to describe the world of the biological molecules we call steroids. I call this vision 'the dance of the steroids'; think of it as action accompanied by music.

Movement 1. Andante con moto
There is a land, near but far away, where busy workers by the millions are doing the work of the body in beautiful, flowing, complex harmony. These are the steroids, turning out products to match our needs, stabilizing, energizing, and nurturing our cells and tissues; ensuring repair and replication of vital body parts; protecting us against damage; and, for a great portion of own adult life, fostering the genesis and development of a new life to carry on the species after our own body ceases to be. The landscape is a hive of hustle and bustle but the prevailing mode is one of synchrony and balance, busy but harmonious. Life is throbbing in a ceaseless flow of energy. We sense the magnitude of activity, the surgings and ebbings of rhythms unseen, and the ungraspable complexity of it all. But at the same time we are aware of order, coordination, and purpose. Despite the complexity and energy apparent, there is an air of majesty and design.

Movement 2. Adagio

A collection of still photographs reveals workers at their benches, bakers busy in their shops, potters at their kilns, carpenters at their labour, homemakers in their nests, firemen at their stations, police standing vigilant, nurses doing their tending, and a host of activities beyond our understanding. At first glance, the workers all look identical. Closer examination reveals slight differences among the various classes of workers. They all seem to be made of the same parts, but with minor variations in how the parts are put together. We see there is no exception, the minor differences among the workers strictly correlates with the work each is doing. Though all are steroids, each is designed with a specific job in mind. What at first appeared to us as chaos is only a fault in our understanding; precision and synchrony are paramount.

Movement 3. Allegro con brio

Live video captures the hustle and bustle of myriad activities; the arrival of raw materials and the departure of finished products; and the ceaseless in-flow of new workers and the out-flow of workers apparently called elsewhere. Just off camera, we are told, are the cholesterol molecules having their parts rearranged to enter the scene as worker units. To our amazement, some workers will, in the blink of an eye, be suddenly transformed from baker to chef, from nurse to fireman, from carpenter to potter without a hint of discontinuity or a missed beat in their activities. Their parts will have been suddenly rearranged and their function switched simultaneously with their newly acquired form. This magical transformation is accomplished by shimmering protein globules (enzymes) passing amongst them, briefly embracing each selected worker molecule and, in a flash of electromagnetic energy, leaving them with slightly altered elements and new function, impressing upon the whole scene a synchrony of design and purpose.

Movement 4. Largo maestoso

Some of the molecules, having reached an end-point in their transformational process, are kept in balanced concentration by being gently swept along in an invisible current to distant parts (the liver) where, their work being done, they are wedded (conjugated) to bile acids and carried silently off our viewing screen. Scientists would say that they are inactivated by hydroxylation (in the case of oestrogens) or hydrogenated and conjugated with glucuronic acid (in the case of progesterone) for excretion in bile. On the periphery of our video scene is a continuous magical influx of new worker units sufficient to meet the rise and fall of their essential functions. In this manner, excesses and/or deficiencies are well prevented and a sense of order pervades, and Figure 2 now fills the screen.

Looking at Figure 2

This flow chart starts in the upper left corner with pregnenolone, having been derived from cholesterol. The flow progresses across through DHEA or down through progesterone leading to metabolic end points appearing at the bottom of the page or along the right-hand margin. These are cortisol, aldosterone, and oestriol. All the other molecules are capable of being converted into some other molecule. Testosterone, for instance, can be a precursor of oestradiol; and androstenedione can be a precursor of either testosterone or oestrone. Oestrone and oestradiol can be interchanged into each other via a redox (reduction/oxidation) system in the liver. Progesterone is a precursor in several pathways; one leading to androstenedione and on to the oestrogens and to testosterone, another to cortisol, and another to corticosterone and aldosterone. Similarly, DHEA is a precursor in the pathway leading to testosterone and androstenedione, the latter leading on to the oestrogens, but not to the corticosteroids.

In addition to their roles as precursors in these steroid biosynthetic pathways, a number of the molecules have specific intrinsic biologic properties of great importance. In Chapter 2, the intrinsic properties and the procreation effects of progesterone were described, and a fuller account will be given in the following chapters. From this graph, however, the pivotal role of progesterone as a steroid precursor is obvious.

Looking at the steroid flow chart, it is clear that, when progesterone is deficient, steroid biosynthesis via the alternative DHEA pathway will be called upon to take up the slack. When this happens, the androgenic steroids along this pathway will become more dominant than when the progesterone pathway pre-dominated. This is the probable cause of the facial hairs and male-pattern scalp hair loss that occurs in elderly women. Evidence of this action is strengthened when replacement of natural progesterone leads, in time, to disappearance of the facial hairs and the restoration of scalp hair.

Recently, the role of dehydroepiandrosterone (DHEA) is arousing interest. In addition to its precursor function in the formation of testosterone and oestrogens, it, too, possesses a spectrum of intrinsic biological effects. It may come as a surprise to many that DHEA is secreted by the adrenal gland in greater doses

Figure 2. Steroidogenesis pathways.

than any of the other adrenal steroids. Yet its function is virtually unknown within the medical profession. As reported by Dr. Alan Gaby[1] in his recent book, *Preventing and Reversing Osteoporosis*, current research suggests that DHEA may be of value in preventing and treating cardiovascular disease, high cholesterol, diabetes, obesity, cancer, Alzheimer's disease, other memory disturbances, immune system disorders, chronic fatigue and ageing. As research progresses, it may be found that DHEA will join progesterone, oestrogen and corticosteroids steroids (and thyroid hormone) as an important hormone in its own right with important benefits when indicated for supplementation.

The continuous cycle of steroid synthesis and their ultimate metabolism is a result of enzyme action monitored and controlled by biofeedback mechanisms originating in the limbic brain (hypothalamus) and evolved over aeons of time. Each arrow in the chart above represents the work of a specific enzyme. The arrow symbol was chosen because it indicates the *direction* of the action. Only in a few instances is an action reversible, as indicated by the double arrows. It is important to realize that enzyme (and hormone) function is dependent on precise molecular configuration and specificity of the molecules involved. Enzymes are amino acid macromolecules continuously created by templates patterned by complex nuclear and mitochondrial chromosomal genomes. They generally require specific vitamin and mineral co-factors for efficient catalyst function. Each enzyme performs but one function, such as the splitting of a single chemical bond in specific molecules for the insertion or deletion of a small molecular fragment, e.g. a hydrogen or oxygen ion or a hydroxyl or other small radical compound. The molecules on which any enzyme may perform their singular function must precisely 'fit', stereochemically and electromagnetically, within the structure of the enzyme. Molecular conformation is the key.

This is the aspect that distinguishes natural steroids most strongly from progestins and other synthetic compounds. With molecular shapes altered by the addition of atoms at unusual positions, synthetic steroids are not subject to the usual metabolic control provided by our enzymes. Thus, their effects can not be 'tuned down' or 'turned off', nor can these synthetic compounds be efficiently excreted by one's usual enzymatic mechanisms. Despite their advertisements, synthetic hormones are *not* equivalent to natural hormones. Harmony and balance, the hallmark of healthy metabolism, are lost when biologically active synthetic compounds (including the xeno-hormones of petrochemical derivation) are thrown into the dance of the steroids. The mischief they can create in the normal ebb and flow of vital steroids should be obvious from the chart in Figure 2.

5

Progesterone and the menstrual cycle

THE HUMAN MENSTRUAL CYCLE has been the subject of scientific investigation since the 1890s. It derives its name from the Greek for 'month' which itself was derived from earlier roots meaning 'moon', i.e. the period of time of the waxing and waning of one new moon to the next. Despite the century of study, full understanding of the menstrual cycle eludes us. Nature is more complex than we can realize.

If one starts at the level of monthly vaginal flow of blood, the hallmark of menstruation, it is known that the female uterus, from puberty to menopause, prepares a specially thickened and blood-filled lining in preparation of possible pregnancy only to shed this lining if pregnancy does not occur in timely fashion; and that this cycle of preparation and shedding occurs at approximately monthly intervals. We know that this uterine cycle is under the control of ovarian-secreted hormones, namely oestrogen and progesterone.

Oestrogen (from 'oestrus' meaning heat or fertility) dominates the first week or so after menstruation, starting the endometrial build-up as the ovarian follicles begin their development of a matured ovum. In addition, oestrogen causes a proliferation of the vaginal mucosa and attendant mucus secretions making it more tolerant of male penetration during sex activity, and increased secretion of the glands of the uterine cervix. Oestrogen is responsible for the changes that take place at puberty in girls, i.e. growth and development of the vagina, uterus, and Fallopian tubes. It causes enlargement of the breasts through growth of ducts, stromal tissue, and the accretion of fat. Oestrogen contributes to molding of female body contours and maturation of the skeleton. It is responsible for the growth of axillary and pubic hair and regional pigmentation of the nipples and areolae.

About twelve days after the beginning of the previous menses, the rising oestrogen (primarily oestradiol) level peaks and then tapers off just as the follicle matures and just before ovulation, after which the follicle becomes the corpus luteum (named so because of its appearance as a small yellow body on the surface of the ovary). The corpus luteum is the site of progesterone production which dominates the second half of the menstrual month, reaching a peak of about 20 mg per day. Progesterone production during the luteal phase of the cycle leads to the development of a secretory endometrium, i.e., more blood-filled in anticipation of a possible fertilized ovum. In addition, progesterone influences the endocervical glands, causing the secretions to change from watery to scant viscid material. (Allowing cervical mucus to dry on a glass slide will allow the appearance of a 'ferning' pattern during oestrogen dominance, not seen during the time of progesterone dominance.) The rise of progesterone at the time of ovulation also has a thermogenic effect, causing a rise of body temperature of about 1 degree Fahrenheit, a finding used to indicate ovulation. If pregnancy does not occur within 10-12 days after ovulation, oestrogen and progesterone levels fall abruptly, triggering the shedding of the accumulated secretory endometrium, i.e. menses, and the cycle begins anew. If pregnancy occurs, progesterone production increases and this shedding of endometrium is prevented, thus preserving the developing embryo. As pregnancy progresses, progesterone production is taken over by the placenta and its secretion increases gradually to levels of 300-400 mg per day during the third trimester.

Thus, the monthly rise and fall of oestrogen and progesterone levels explain the events of menstruation. But what determines the synchronous cycling of these two gonadal hormones? This, it turns out, is controlled by two hormones secreted by the anterior pituitary, i.e. the gonadotropic hormones follicle stimulating hormone (FSH) and luteinizing hormone (LH). Simply put, FSH drives the ovary to make oestrogen, promotes maturation of the follicle, and, at the same time, sensitizes the follicle receptors to LH ; whereas, LH rises a day or two before ovulation, peaking just as ovulation gets underway, and then falls dramatically as the corpus luteum starts turning out progesterone.

Now the question becomes: what determines the marvellous synchrony of FSH and LH? The answer lies in the hypothalamus, within the limbic brain. This marvellous neural nucleus, situated in the brain just above the pituitary, monitors not only the serum levels of oestrogen and progesterone but also the various body effects they are creating, and, with exquisite timing, produces and sends to the pituitary (via special vein-like channels) a peptide hormone made of ten linked amino acids called gonadotropin-releasing hormone

(GnRH) which is responsible for the release of either or both of the gonadotropins, FSH and LH. At the present, it is not known how a single hypothalamic hormone can control both FSH and LH. The varying blood concentrations of each suggests either (1) another regulatory hormone or (2) complex feedback effects of sex steroids and perhaps other unknown gonadal factors on the pituitary and/or hypothalamus to explain the divergent patterns of release of each gonadotropin.

As might be imagined, the complete mechanism of the action of this vital nucleus within the hypothalamus is beyond present knowledge. It might help, however, to realize that the limbic brain, of which the hypothalamus is a part, is a bio-feedback information and control centre with multiple neural centres sharing and integrating myriad biochemical, hormonal, immunologic, and emotional conditions. It functions as a giant analog computer complex with the capacity to formulate and send messenger peptides to the pituitary as well as to control our autonomic nervous system balance and immuno-modulators, and creates for us our sense of emotions and their physiologic responses. When all this is grasped sufficiently, it is no wonder that menstruation (and a great number of other things) can be affected by emotional states of mind, stress, diet, other hormones (e.g., thyroid), illness, or drugs of all sorts.

Clearly, this is a system one would not prefer to have tampered with. Yet, this is what happens when progestins are prescribed. With the various pituitary and hypothalamic gonadal hormone receptors filled with synthetically altered hormones, as in contraception pills, the net result is inhibition of one's natural hormones. In the past, some of these drugs resulted in permanent loss of ovary function ('secondary amenorrhoea'), much to the consternation of, or possibly a tragedy for, the woman who had used them. The long lists of potential side effects for each and every one of the progestins does not seem to deter their use. And last but not least, the inhibition of progesterone and its multiple benefits described in Chapter 2 is not presently being addressed by patients' physicians. Progesterone is a major player in the normal functioning of the menstrual cycle. Its loss surely becomes manifest as disease. The confusion wrought within the hypothalamus by the absence of the true hormones will reverberate throughout the neuro-immuno-endocrinologic province of this remarkable limbic centre with effects that are bound not to be recognized by one's physician.

There is also the problem of anovulatory cycles. For reasons yet to be explained, a good proportion of women in their thirties (and some even earlier) and long before actual menopause, will, on occasion, not ovulate during their menstrual month.[1,2] Without ovulation, no corpus luteum results and no progesterone is made. Several problems can result form this. One is the month-long presence of unopposed oestrogen with all its attendant side effects leading to the syndrome known as PMS. Another is the present, generally unrecognized, problem of progesterone's role in osteoporosis. Contemporary medicine is still unaware that progesterone stimulates osteoblast-mediated new bone formation.[3] Both of these topics will be addressed in chapters that follow. A third is the inter-relationship between progesterone loss and stress. Stress influences limbic brain function including the functioning of the hypothalamus. In brief, stress (and a bad diet) can induce anovulatory cycles. The consequent lack of progesterone interferes with adrenal corticosteroids by which one normally responds to stress. The effects of stress, therefore, are heightened, predisposing one to anovulatory cycles, the ultimate vicious cycle. This, too, will be discussed in a chapter to follow.

Given the complexity and heterogenicity of cause and effect in the intricate arrangement of stress, diet, hypothalamic and pituitary function, and normal hormones, the prevailing attitude that female health concerns are merely a matter of hormone 'deficiency' is vastly overstating the case. Women are right to be upset with their doctors.

Steps in reproductive hormone cycle

(Numbered steps refer to Figure 3 opposite.)

1 Low levels of oestrogen and progesterone stimulate the hypothalamus to send *gonadotropin releasing hormone* (GnRH) to the pituitary.
2 Stimulated by GnRH, the pituitary sends *follicle stimulating hormone* (FSH) to the ovary. Ovary follicles produce *oestrogen* while they mature. In about 10 days the high oestrogen level signals the pituitary production of *luteinizing hormone* (LH) for ovulation.
3 Prior to ovulation *oestrogen* is the dominant gonadal hormone. After ovulation the follicle becomes the corpus luteum, producing *progesterone* which becomes the dominant gonadal hormone during the second two weeks of the menstrual cycle.
4 The oestrogen-mediated proliferative endometrium changes to secretory endometrium by progesterone. When the corpus luteum involutes and both oestrogen and progesterone levels fall, the endometrial lining is shed.

Figure 3. Steps in reproductive hormone cycle.

5   Serum oestrogen and progesterone levels rise and fall as described in steps 2-4.

6   Oestrogen and progesterone are metabolized in liver and excreted in bile and urine.

7   Serum oestrogen and progesterone levels are monitored by the hypothalamus.

6

Progesterone and pregnancy

WOMEN NEED to be very, very wary of what conventional medicine has to offer, and *physicians need to dare to listen to their patients and question the prevailing dogmas.* In no area of medicine is this more true than fertility treatments: most often the simple, obvious questions are not asked, and the simple, obvious (and inexpensive) treatments are not given.

Getting pregnant and staying pregnant

You can try this at home

There's no question that more women than ever are having problems conceiving, and that more women are being required to become familiar with the complex issues of infertility in order to become pregnant. The other increasingly common problem of pregnancy is miscarriage: one in three pregnancies in the U.S. ends in miscarriage.

I'm going to give you some simple solutions you can try at home that may help prevent a miscarriage. But first I want to tell you a little bit about your eggs, follicles and cycles, and why you may be having trouble conceiving.

Popping an egg

A molecular biologist friend of mine refers to ovulation as 'popping an egg.' This is a good metaphor for ovulation, because a combination of hormonal and chemical messages in the brain and the ovary all need to coordinate and coalesce at the right moments in the menstrual cycle in order for an ovarian follicle to get the message to mature and 'pop' out of the ovary, where it releases the egg into the fallopian tube.

Ovulation is the first requirement for pregnancy, but we can't take it for granted, even in young women. As reported by Peter Ellison of Harvard, a study of 19 presumably healthy premenopausal women with a mean age of 29 found that six of them — or 31% — failed to ovulate at any time during their menstrual cycle.[1]

When women do ovulate, it doesn't necessarily occur within the narrow time boundaries dictated by traditional medicine. The advent of the saliva hormone assay has significantly broadened our understanding of the timing of ovulation. When salivary testing is done throughout a woman's menstrual cycle, several stunning observations can be made.

For example, ovulation in normal women occurs at almost any time of the menstrual cycle, but most commonly from day 5 to day 15, rather than from day 12 to 14, as most textbooks say.

Salivary testing also reveals that the ovulatory surge of progesterone that occurs after ovulation is lasting for only two to four days in some women, rather than the normal 10 to 12. This means that something is wrong, because adequate progesterone levels are crucial for proper implantation of the egg in the endometrium (the uterine lining) as well as for the survival of the fertilised egg. A fall in progesterone after only two to four days would eliminate the implantation or survival of any fertilised egg.

The life and times of your follicles

Strange as it might seem, ovaries and testes are formed early in the life of the embryo. By the third week, more than 500,000 follicles are being formed in the embryo's ovary, and each follicle supposedly contains an ovum (egg) awaiting full development after puberty. (In males, the equivalent case concerns Sertoli cells in the testes.) Any of these follicles, upon ovulation, becomes the corpus luteum that produces the progesterone necessary for the survival of the fertilised egg.

Exposure to pesticides or other petrochemical xenobiotics (environmental substances with hormonal effects) during the embryonic period is particularly damaging to the development of ovaries. (For details, read *Our Stolen Future* by Theo Colborn et al., Penguin Books, 1997.) That is, the mother may not show toxic effects to minute doses of these toxins, but the embryo is exquisitely sensitive to them. If the embryo is female, her ovarian follicles may be damaged.

These effects have serious consequences. Damaged or dysfunctional follicles will not be able to pop an egg or produce sufficient progesterone later in life. The incidence of progesterone deficiency among women aged 35 in the industrialised world is about 50%. Treatment with progesterone is helpful but not necessarily curative for this condition. Dysfunctional follicles, which cause progesterone deficiency, lead to ovarian cysts. These cysts will usually clear up after proper progesterone levels are restored, but the ovary still may not be able to produce a viable egg. It is also follicle dysfunction which causes many early miscarriages.

What you can do about miscarriage

Although there's nothing we can do about a follicle that can't pop an egg, miscarriages caused by 'luteal phase failure' — in which the follicles ovulate normally but fail to continue their progesterone production at levels necessary for successful implantation of the fertilised egg and development of the embryo — can be prevented by progesterone treatment. I encounter women with this problem all the time.

At one of my talks, a woman told me she was having difficulty having a baby. She had a four-year-old son, and had been pregnant several times since then, but each pregnancy resulted in an early miscarriage. Repeated early miscarriages are often caused by luteal phase failure. The problem is common and is occurring in younger and younger women, probably because of embryonic exposure to xenobiotics. These women do not have trouble getting pregnant: their problem is getting the embryo to survive and not miscarry.

What should they do? They need to increase and maintain their progesterone levels to the point where they can support their pregnancy, and they can do this by supplementing with progesterone. Normally, when an egg is fertilised, this sends chemical messages that cause the follicle to increase its production of progesterone to 30 to 40 mg per day, double or triple what it made during the luteal phase of the monthly cycle when the woman was not pregnant. The level of progesterone increases gradually until well into the third month of pregnancy. By that time, the placenta is well developed and is producing progressively more progesterone within the uterus. By the third trimester (the final three months of the pregnancy) progesterone production reaches 300 to 350 mg/day, more than 20 times higher than normal.

Correcting luteal phase failure

When supplementing progesterone for luteal phase failure, conventional physicians often use injectable progesterone or vaginal progesterone suppositories in doses of several hundred mg/day. They give so much in order to produce serum levels of progesterone similar to levels in the early pregnancy. But serum levels of progesterone are misleading. Most conventional physicians do not know that 90% of bioavailable progesterone is carried by red blood cells and not in the blood serum (see Chapter 14). Progesterone in the blood serum is protein-bound and less than 10 per cent is bioavailable. Because of this simple lack of understanding, conventional medicine routinely gives excessive doses of progesterone to patients with luteal phase failure in order to raise serum progesterone levels. As a result, the success rates for this approach are usually less than 30%.

It is much more effective to supplement with transdermal natural progesterone, which is carried in a bioavailable fashion by the red blood cells after absorption. Progesterone creams can easily supply the proper dose of 30 to 40 mg/day, or more if needed. The creams I usually recommend provide 450 to 500 mg of progesterone per ounce. One-quarter of a teaspoon of cream supplies about 20 mg. This dose can be applied at bedtime and in the morning to provide 40 mg per day. For this use, I recommend avoiding creams with wild yam (diosgenin), herbs or other active ingredients.

As soon as pregnancy is confirmed by a blood test, a woman at risk for miscarriage should start using a progesterone cream that supplies that dosage. (Women who are already using progesterone cream should simply continue if they become pregnant, and increase the dose.) After the first month of pregnancy, the dose can be increased gradually to 60 to 80 mg/day.

After the third month of pregnancy, progesterone production in the placenta increases so much that, in theory, supplemental progesterone becomes less important. However, most of my patients felt more comfortable continuing the cream throughout pregnancy, and stopping one week before their expected delivery date.

At that time the baby triggers its own delivery by excreting cortisol in its urine. This reduces progesterone's uterine effects, and allows uterine contractions. In the mother's body, the steep fall in progesterone that occurs with delivery stimulates the production of the hormone prolactin, which stimulates the production of milk. Women who suffer from postpartum depression often find relief when they use a little bit of natural progesterone cream.

Thus it is clear why progesterone is the progestational hormone: its presence at the proper time and in the proper amounts is essential to conception and maintaining a healthy pregnancy.

Some possible causes of the inability to conceive

Some of the more common underlying causes of the inability to conceive (excluding problems with the sperm) could include the following:

- Mechanical obstructions (blocked Fallopian tubes)
- Hormone problems (e.g. hypothyroidism)
- Primary ovary failure (ovaries fail to develop)
- Secondary ovarian failure (e.g. after years of birth control pills)

- Improper timing of intercourse (the presumption that ovulation only occurs at days 12 to 14 of the menstrual cycle is erroneous)
- Toxicity (fertility rates inversely correlate with fluoride exposure, for example)
- Genetic (Turner's syndrome for example)
- Stress (stress-induced anovulatory — non-ovulating — periods are common)
- Nutritional (anorexia: starvation routinely limits fertility)

The list of possible causes of infertility is actually much longer than this. Achieving successful pregnancy is a precarious thing; experts think that one-third of all fertilized eggs fail to survive.

7

Progesterone and menopause

A H, MENOPAUSE — Nature's course correction when a woman no longer has to put up with the nuisance of monthly periods, free to exercise her lusty libido without the risk of pregnancy and the burden of bearing children, a time when she is likely freed of child care, still in good health, and full of the wisdom of life. What a blessed gift of mother Nature!

Wait a minute. Is that the same menopause we perceive as the bench mark of life when fertility is over, unpredictable hot flushes and mood swings abound, vaginal dryness and fibroids become conversation pieces among female friends, cancer risks rise, bones deteriorate and osteoporotic fractures loom, and life enters a downward spiral to old age and infirmity? What a bummer!

Such diverse views bring to mind the old story about the politician being asked his view on alcohol use. He responds that he will be only too glad to answer the question but first he wants to know whether the questioner has in mind the alcohol that helps soothe one's daily troubles, that lubricates social intercourse and is shared at joyous occasions, or does the questioner have in mind the alcohol that befuddles the mind, poisons the body, causes a man to lose his job and forget his family responsibilities, and leads one to degradation and disgrace. Tell me which alcohol you mean, he says, and I'll tell you how I feel about it.

Or, recall the picture in psychology books of what can appear to be either a vase or a silhouette view of two faces nose-to-nose. Both views can be clearly seen but not at the same time. In the case of menopause, how can the two views be reconciled?

It is helpful sometimes to ask the question: Did mother Nature make a mistake in designing women such that life after menopause is so doleful, or that a woman's life after her fertile years has no future except to deteriorate and die? If one holds to the faith that mother Nature does not make mistakes like that, one can than ask if perhaps the present problems we are having with menopause are due to some mistake we are making, not mother Nature. Let us look again at menopause.

There is a common misconception that menopause, the cessation of menses, means that a woman no longer makes female hormones, that she needs oestrogen replacement and the continual care of a doctor; that she has a deficiency disease. The truth is that she merely makes less oestrogen than is necessary for the monthly preparation of her endometrium for pregnancy. Oestrogen does not fall to zero; her body still makes oestrogen from androstenedione in her fat cells.

Progesterone levels, on the other hand, do fall to zero, or very close to it, with menopause or even for some time before menopause. Serum levels of progesterone in menopausal women are lower than that of a man's. As we have seen, progesterone is a major precursor of corticosteroids. There is, however, an alternative pathway via dehydroepiandrosterone (DHEA). In the absence of progesterone, the body can increase DHEA which leads to androstenedione and on to oestrogen and corticosteroid synthesis. As oestrogen levels fall with menopause, the androgenic properties of androstenedione become operative, leading to facial and body hair (hirsutism) and male pattern baldness. It has been noted by others that little old women come to look like little old men. Supplementation with natural progesterone is obviously the treatment of choice.

A progesterone vignette

I am reminded of a menopausal woman in Canada who sent to me a 10-lb packet of her medical records from the 5 or 6 doctors she had consulted, asking for my advice. In the packet was a series of laboratory tests for serum progesterone. The patient had been put on the progestin, medroxyprogesterone acetate (Provera), and her doctor had ordered a serum progesterone level. Finding it still zero, he doubled the progestin dose and ordered a second test. This, too, was zero. He doubled the progestin dose again and ordered a third test which again indicated zero progesterone. But on this lab report, the technician had written, 'Doctor, you are giving this lady Provera. You are ordering tests for serum progesterone. Provera is not progesterone!' By this time, the patient was experiencing numerous side effects from the drug, specifically loss of appetite, nausea, indigestion, fatigue and depression. I circled the lab tech's comment in red and sent it back to the lady with an information sheet on natural progesterone. Several months later I got a very nice note from the lady telling me how much better she felt using natural progesterone and that she had fired all but one of her doctors. She had also included a generous cheque though I had made no charge.

• • •

To reiterate, oestrogen levels do not fall to zero at menopause. If this is so, you ask, why do some women suffer from vaginal dryness, uterine fibroids, an increased risk of breast and uterine cancer, hot flushes, and dry, wrinkly skin when menopause occurs? The answer lies in a number of factors, not the least of which has to do with progesterone.

One of the paradoxes in female hormone physiology is that oestrogen and progesterone, though mutually antagonistic in some of their effects, each sensitize receptor sites for the other. That is, the presence of oestrogen makes body target tissues more sensitive to progesterone and the presence of progesterone does the same for oestrogen. Each sets the stage for the body to be more responsive to the other; an interesting example of nature's efficiency.

A peculiarity of industrialised societies is the prevalence of uterine fibroids, breast and/or uterine cancer, fibrocystic breasts, PMS, and premenopausal bone loss as well as a high incidence of postmenopausal osteoporosis. If oestrogen loss is the major hormonal factor in female osteoporosis, for example, why should significant bone loss occur during the 10-15 years before menopause? It is a fact that, in the US, peak bone mass in women occurs in the mid-thirties and that a good percentage of women arrive at menopause with osteoporosis well underway. Further, it is known that uterine fibroids atrophy after the menopausal decline of oestrogen; that fibrocystic breasts are made worse by oestrogen supplementation and easily treated by progesterone; that breast and/or uterine cancer risk is increased by oestrogen and largely prevented by progesterone; and that PMS can often be successfully treated by natural progesterone.

The common thread running through all these conditions is oestrogen dominance secondary to a relative insufficiency of progesterone. How can this happen in menstruating women? It happens when women have anovulatory cycles. As we have seen, progesterone is produced by the corpus luteum, itself formed at the time of ovulation. Anovulatory cycles may be regular or irregular though often the woman discerns a different pattern in the menstrual flow, i.e., heavier or longer. If anovulation is suspected (and usually it is not), it can be revealed by testing for low serum progesterone levels during days 18-26 of the menstrual cycle.

The point of this brief detour is that low premenopausal progesterone, as a consequence of anovulatory cycles, can induce increased oestrogen levels and lead to symptomatically significant oestrogen dominance prior to menopause. The most common age for breast or uterine cancer to originate is five years before menopause (though it may not be diagnosed for eight to ten years). And there is more. The hypothalamic biofeedback mechanisms activated by this lack of progesterone as a woman approaches menopause, leads to elevation of GnRH and pituitary release of FSH and LH. Potential consequences of this are increased oestrogen production, loss of corticosteroid production, and intracellular edema. Heightened activity of the hypothalamus, a component of the limbic brain, can induce hyperactivity of adjacent limbic nuclei leading to mood swings, fatigue, feelings of being cold, and inappropriate responses to other stressors. Not uncommonly, hypothyroidism is suspected despite normal thyroid hormone levels.

Around age 45-50, sometimes a little earlier or later, oestrogen levels fall and the menstrual flow becomes less and/or irregular and eventually ceases. Oestrogen levels have fallen below that necessary for endometrial stimulation. In most other cultures, this event is otherwise symptomless. In the US, menopause is relatively symptom-free in 50-60% of women. The rest, however, experience hot flushes, mood swings, vaginal dryness, and a distressing growth of facial and body hair. During the months when menses were merely irregular, FSH levels tend to rise and to fluctuate considerably. This is called the perimenopausal stage. With actual menopause, FSH and LH levels rise as the menopausal decline in oestrogen diminishes the negative feedback effect on the pituitary. Ovarian failure may occur at any age, but menopause prior to age 40 is considered premature.

The failure of the ovary to respond to gonadotropin hormones is due to a final depletion of oocytes and the surrounding follicle cells. Of the millions of oocytes present before birth, approximately 300,000 are present at menarche (puberty). Subsequently, hundreds vanish every cycle, including the cycles induced by hormonal contraception. Eventually, at menopause, the supply is reduced to only about 1000 follicles which is insufficient to sustain the cyclic hormonal process necessary for menstruation. Thus, it is the disappearance of oocytes and follicle cells rather than age, per se, that causes menopause.[1]

Fertility is a also a function of the number of follicles. Regardless of coital frequency, the monthly probability of a 38-year-old woman conceiving and carrying to term is only about one-quarter that in a woman under age 30.[2]

Further, it is a fact that conception after the age of 35 or so is attended by an increased likelihood of congenital deformities,[3] e.g., Down's syndrome, secondary to imperfect gamete (ova) production. It should be clear that proper nutrition and avoidance of toxins damaging to oocytes should be high on anyone's list of priorities in life.

We have now come to the crux of the problem. Healthy, well nourished follicle cells produce a healthy balance of oestrogen and progesterone. Follicle cell dysfunction from any cause, especially from intracellular nutritional deficiencies and/or toxins, will lead to progesterone deficiency and oestrogen dominance combined with elevated FSH and LH levels and hypothalamic hyperactivity. The net result, of course, is the gamut of hormone imbalance symptoms seen in peri-menopausal and menopausal women daily in doctors' offices. Women's self-help groups, menopause books, and lay magazine articles attest to the prevalence of this disorder. The question now is — what ought to (or can) be done about it?

The answer, of course, is good nutrition, avoidance of toxins, and the proper supplementation, when indicated for hormone balance, of real, honest-to-God, natural progesterone.

Good nutrition means plenty of fresh vegetables, whole grains, and fruit eaten as unprocessed as possible and uncontaminated by insecticides, artificial colouring agents or preservatives, or other toxic ingredients. Given the present methods of meat production, these should be minimised. Eggs are probably fine, as well as are modest servings of ocean fish and fowl (most insecticides are fat soluble and found primarily in the skin of fowl and fish). Vegetable and seed oils obtained by high-pressure squeezing should be avoided because of the problem of *trans*-fatty acids. Olive oil does not require such high-pressure squeezing and is OK. Flaxseed oil, walnut oil, Evening Primrose oil, and pumpkin oil are all especially nutritious because of their complement of essential fatty acids (i.e., linoleic acid and α-linolenic acid). Due to the pervasiveness of our processed food diet, a limited number of nutrients should be supplemented: vitamin C, 1 gram twice a day; vitamin E, 400 iu/day); betacarotene, 15 mg/day; zinc 15-30 mg/day; and magnesium 100-300 mg/day. Cigarette smoking is not allowed and alcohol consumption should be strictly limited.

Supplementation with natural progesterone is a clinical decision based on signs and symptoms of oestrogen dominance, listed below. (See also pp49-50.)

Signs and symptoms of oestrogen dominance

- water retention, edema
- breast swelling, fibrocystic breasts
- premenstrual mood swings, depression
- loss of libido
- heavy or irregular menses
- uterine fibroid
- craving for sweets
- weight gain, fat deposition at hips and thighs

If progesterone supplementation is decided upon for a perimenopausal woman, one can choose among capsules, sublingual drops, and transdermal cream. Over the years, my patients have generally opted for the transdermal cream because of its skin benefits (it is an excellent skin moisturizer), low cost, and ease of application. The usual cream contains a bit over 475 mg/ounce (960 mg in a 2-oz jar). Since normal progesterone production by the corpus luteum can reach 20 mg/day between days 18 and 26 of the cycle, I usually recommend using one ounce of the cream between day 12 and day 26 to approximate normal levels. The actual dose is determined by the response obtained, i.e. relief of symptoms. Some patients have found the two-ounce jar to be preferable. Since natural progesterone is notable for its freedom from side effects, such latitude in dosing carries no risk. Stopping the cream at day 26 usually results in a normal menses within 48 hours or so.

Postmenopausal women not receiving oestrogen supplementation have an even wider latitude in using progesterone cream. They may choose, for convenience, to select a dosage schedule based on the calendar month. The cream may be applied over a 24-25 day time period and then discontinued until the next month. A short period of not using the hormone tends to maintain receptor sensitivity.

Postmenopausal women receiving a cyclic oestrogen supplement should reduce their dosage to one-half when starting the progesterone. (Progesterone enhances receptor sensitivity of oestrogen.) If they do not, they are likely to experience symptoms of oestrogen dominance the first one to two months of progesterone use. Alternatively, the cream may be applied during the latter two weeks of oestrogen use and both hormones discontinued for one week each month.

Many postmenopausal women do not need oestrogen supplements. Not only does a woman's body continue to produce some oestrogen but she is ingesting phytooestrogens (oestrogenic substances found in plants) and is exposed to xenooestrogens (oestrogenic substances of petrochemical origin in the environment). The addition of progesterone enhances the receptors of oestrogen and thus her 'need' for oestrogen may not exist. If neither vaginal dryness nor hot flushes are present after three months of progesterone therapy, it is unlikely that oestrogen supplements are needed.

Hot flushes are not a sign of oestrogen deficiency *per se*, but are due to heightened hypothalamic activity (vasomotor lability) secondary to low levels of oestrogen and progesterone which, if raised, would produce a negative feedback effect to the pituitary and hypothalamus. Once progesterone levels are raised, oestrogen receptors in these areas become more sensitive, and hot flushes usually subside. The validity of this mechanism can be tested by measuring FSH and LH levels before and after adequate progesterone supplementation.

Why does progesterone deficiency occur?

The final question to be answered is: why does progesterone deficiency occur? Did mother Nature make a mistake? Mother Nature did not make the mistake; we did. Just as with phytooestrogens, many (over 5000 known) plants make sterols that are progestogenic. In cultures whose diets are rich in fresh vegetables of all sorts, progesterone deficiency does not exist. Not only do the women of these cultures have healthy ovaries with healthy follicles producing sufficient progesterone, but, at menopause, their diets provide sufficient progestogenic substances to keep their libido high, their bones strong, and their passage through menopause uneventful and symptom-free. Our food supply system uses many processed foods and foods that are picked days before being sold. Their vitamin (especially vitamin C) content falls and their sterol levels fall. We do not receive the progestogenic substances our forebears did. A recent *Lancet* report of bone mineral density results of bones in bodies buried almost 300 years ago in England showed better bones at all ages compared to our skeletons of today. It is likely that both exercise and diet had something to do with that.

Progesterone can also be extracted from placentas obtained at deliveries. This is the practice in Europe. Worldwide, however, the most common source of natural progesterone is the wild yam, grown for the purpose. Yam produces the sterol, diosgenin, which is quite easily converted to natural progesterone. Diets high in yam consumption (e.g., as by the Trobriand islanders) provide sufficient progesterone to prevent the sort of problems discussed in this chapter. Further, traditional practices among many cultures provide relief of these problems by the use of herbs, such as Dong Quai, Black Cohosh, and Fennel, which contain active oestrogenic and progestogenic substances.

In western industrialized cultures, pharmaceutical companies buy natural progesterone (derived from yams) and then chemically alter its molecular form to produce the various progestins, which, being *not* found in nature, are patentable and therefore more profitable. Most physicians are unaware (1) that their prescription progestins are made from progesterone (from yams), and (2) that natural progesterone is available, safer than progestins, more effective, and relatively inexpensive.

The secret for the successful management of menopausal symptoms is natural progesterone.

8

A word about oestrogen

A S SHOULD BE CLEAR BY NOW, progesterone and oestrogen are closely inter-related in many ways. Progesterone is a precursor in the normal biosynthetic pathway for oestrogen; they are, in many instances, antagonistic; and each sensitizes receptors for the other. Therefore, our understanding of progesterone will be enhanced if we understand oestrogen a bit better.

First, there is a semantic problem to clear up. As related in Chapter 1, the early researchers found evidence of an oestrus-producing hormone (i.e., oestrogen) and then, in 1929, Corner and Allen established the existence of a corpus luteum hormone necessary for the successful promotion of gestation (i.e., progesterone). Then, oestrogen was found to be not one hormone but a group of similar hormones of varying degrees of activity, all made by the ovary. Each, as they were found, was given a specific chemical name and the word 'oestrogen' became the name of the *class* of hormones with oestrus activity. The three most important hormones of this oestrogen class are oestrone, oestradiol, and oestriol. In popular writing, however, each of the specific members of the class continues to be referred to as oestrogen. In the case of progesterone, only a single hormone is found. Thus, 'progesterone' is both the name of the class and of the single member of the class.

Later, when plant extractions were found to have progestational activity and, even later, when synthetic versions with progestational activity were created, various authors described them as 'progestins', or 'gestogens', or 'progestagens'. Unfortunately, in the pharmaceutical promotion that followed, the word 'progesterone' was also used to describe these other compounds with the ability to sustain the human secretory endometrium, despite their many side effects (not found in progesterone) and the lack of many of the other abilities of natural progesterone as produced by the corpus luteum. This confusion still exists in the minds of many physicians and writers. Gail Sheehy, in her popular 1991 book *The Silent Passage*, for instance, admits to being so confused about the names that she decided to call all of them 'progesterone' throughout the book even though she is generally writing about the synthetic progestins.[1]

The word 'oestrogen' generally refers to the class of hormones produced by the body with somewhat similar oestrus-like actions. Phytooestrogens refer to plant compounds with oestrogen-like activity; and xenooestrogens refer to other environmental compounds (usually petrochemical) with oestrogen-like activity.

The compound, p - Anol, is an active oestrogenic agent found in fennel and anise. Diethylstilboestrol (DES), which resembles two molecules of p - Anol linked end to end, is fully as potent as the most active gonadal hormone, oestradiol. It can be inexpensively synthesized and is highly active when taken orally. In the past it was used for regulation of the menstrual cycle, in contraceptives, and to prevent premature labour. However, it has been implicated in certain types of cancer (e.g., cervical cancer in daughters of mothers who were given DES during pregnancy) and its use has been superseded by other, presumably less dangerous, compounds. DES was also used most extensively in beef cattle to fatten them up more quickly for slaughter.

A common feature of oestrogenic compounds is the phenolated A-ring of the molecule. This molecular configuration of a phenolated A-ring, as in oestrogens, is not present among progesterone, testosterone, and corticosterone molecules. Most likely, this difference is the reason for oestrogen's different receptor specificity and physiologic actions. Phenolic compounds are common among petrochemical derivatives which are pervasively polluting our environment. Some of these are extremely potent oestrogenic compounds (called xenooestrogens), even at nanogram doses. Known xenooestrogens include plant-produced coumetrol, equol, tetrahydrocannabinol, zearalenone; pesticides such as DDT and kepone; and a combustion by-product, 3,9-D-dihydroxybenz [a] anthracene.[2] This unrecognized exposure to oestrogenic compounds may possibly be a significant causal factor in the breast cancer and the recently identified decline in male sperm production.[3]

Oestrogen synthesis

Because of their respective position in the biosynthetic pathway, oestrone is referred to as E_1, oestradiol as E_2, and oestriol as E_3. In the non-pregnancy state, E_1 and E_2 are produced by the ovary in microgram quantities and E_3 is only a scant by-product of E_1 metabolism. Relative serum E_1 and E_2 levels are determined less by their synthesis rate than by a reversible liver redox system which can convert one into the other and results in higher levels of E_2.

During pregnancy, however, the placenta is the major source of oestrogens;

E_3 is produced in milligram quantities while E_1 and E_2 are produced in microgram amounts. E_2 excretion now becomes least. Instead of de novo synthesis from acetate via cholesterol, pregnenalone, or progesterone, placental E_3 synthesis requires DHEA obtained from DHEA-S (sulphated DHEA) of either maternal or foetal (adrenal) origin. Because of foetal participation in E_3 formation, serum E_3 measurements can be a sensitive clinical indicator of placenta and/or foetal status.

The placenta also becomes the major source of progesterone, producing 300-400 milligrams per day during the third trimester. Oestriol (E_3) and progesterone, therefore, are the major sex steroids during pregnancy. Both oestriol and progesterone are essentially devoid of the ability to affect secondary sex characteristics and thus the sexual development of the foetus is determined solely by its own DNA and not the sex hormones of the mother. Lurking as an unknown factor in the later development of one's sexual preference is the possibility of influence by the xenooestrogens of our petrochemically polluted environment.

Among the three oestrogens, oestradiol is most stimulating to the breast and oestriol is the least; their relative ratio of activity being 1000:1.[4] Studies of two decades ago found oestradiol (and oestrone to a lesser extent) to increase one's risk of breast cancer whereas oestriol is protective.[5] Synthetic ethinyloestradiol, commonly used in oestrogen supplements and contraceptives, is even more of a risk because of high oral absorption and slow metabolism and excretion. Since this factor of slow metabolism and excretion is true of all synthetic oestrogens, one would think that, in all cases of oestrogen supplementation, the natural hormones would be superior.

Conversely, oestriol is the oestrogen most active on the vagina, cervix and vulva. In cases of postmenopausal vaginal dryness and atrophy which predisposes a woman to vaginitis and cystitis, oestriol supplementation would theoretically be the most effective (and safest) oestrogen to use.[6]

Oestrogen effects

Teleologically, oestrogen might be thought of in terms of procreation and survival of the foetus. It would seem advantageous to the baby for the expectant mother to be able, in times of famine, to store body fat. Thus, the effects of oestrogen include far more than merely its action on creating the female body form and its stimulation of the uterus and breasts. During times of consistent dietary abundance, oestrogen's effects are potentially deleterious.

It is worthwhile to compare the physiological effects of oestrogen and progesterone.

Oestrogen effects	Progesterone effects
creates proliferative endometrium	maintains secretory endometrium
breast stimulation	protects against breast fibrocysts
increased body fat	helps use fat for energy
salt and fluid retention	natural diuretic
depression and headaches	natural anti-depressant
interferes with thyroid hormone	facilitates thyroid hormone action
increased blood clotting	normalizes blood clotting
decreases libido	restores libido
impairs blood sugar control	normalizes blood sugar levels
loss of zinc and retention of copper	normalizes zinc and copper levels
reduced oxygen levels in all cells	restores proper cell oxygen levels
increased risk of endometrial cancer	prevents endometrial cancer
increased risk of breast cancer	helps prevent breast cancer
slightly restrains osteoclast function	stimulates osteoblast bone building
reduces vascular tone	necessary for survival of embryo
	precursor of corticosterone production

Oestrogen dominance (unopposed oestrogen)

It is clear that, no matter how valuable, oestrogen, when unopposed by progesterone, is not something wholly to be desired. Stated differently, it is clear that many of oestrogen's undesirable side effects are effectively prevented by progesterone. I would propose that a new syndrome be recognized: that of *oestrogen dominance*, whether it occurs as a result of exogenous oestrogen given postmenopausally or during the premenopausal anovulatory phase so common these days. Unfortunately, it is the custom of contemporary medicine to prescribe oestrogen alone for women without intact uteri and, equally unfortunate, premenopausal oestrogen dominance is simply ignored.

The most common reason offered for postmenopausal women to take oestrogen is protection against osteoporosis. Here the picture is quite clear; oestrogen lack stimulates the osteoclast bone cells to increased bone resorption. However, this effect fades in 5 years or so and, thereafter, bone loss continues at the same pace as in those women not using oestrogen.[7] The more important factor in osteoporosis is the lack of progesterone which causes a *decrease* in osteoblast-mediated new bone formation. This will be discussed more fully in Chapter 11.

See also 'Signs of oestrogen dominance', pp44-45.

Some guidelines for supplementing safely and effectively

Here's a story that I hear every day: Joan, a premenopausal woman in her mid-40s goes to her doctor complaining of hot flushes, poor sleep, and lack of energy. She is still having regular periods. Her doctor tests her oestradiol, FSH, LH, and progesterone levels, and finds them all to be normal except for very low progesterone. He then prescribes oestradiol supplementation! Within three months Joan gains 25 pounds, is sleeping even less, feels irritable and anxious, and has headaches.

Another oestrogen supplementation scenario that I hear every day is the woman who is prescribed oestrogen alone (without progesterone) and within a year has a pap smear that shows cervical dysplasia, soon followed by a hysterectomy. I consider this medical malpractice, but it happens to hundreds of women every day.

Confusion reigns on the subject of oestrogen replacement: What time of life? How much? Which kind? How often? Is it safe?

Here are some fairly simple guidelines to help you make your own educated decisions. The two most important basic guidelines in oestrogen supplementation are:

1   Only women who are clearly deficient in oestrogen should take it.
2   Oestrogen should always be taken with progesterone regardless of your age or whether you have a uterus.

It's that simple, but these guidelines are routinely ignored by conventional medicine. It's almost certain that a woman around the age of 50 who visits her doctor will receive a prescription for oestrogen regardless of symptoms, and often without even a blood test.

Conventional medicine also fails to discriminate between different oestrogens whether natural or synthetic, phytooestrogens, horse oestrogen or human. They fail to consider the interaction between oestrogen and diet, or oestrogen and progesterone, let alone its interrelationship to testosterone, other androgens, thyroid, or corticosteroids.

Another issue I have with oestrogen supplementation in conventional medicine is gross overdosing. For decades I have been suggesting that women who need oestrogen take only half or a quarter of the usual recommended dosages.

A recent study[8] supports this point of view. In a group of women 65 to 80 years of age who had never used hormone replacement therapy of any kind, blood levels of oestradiol (one of the human oestrogens) were measured. It was found that two-thirds of these women had blood serurm oestradiol levels greater than 5 pg/ml, a level consistent with optimal bone benefit. In the one-third of women who had oestradiol levels lower than 5 pg/ml, the oestrogen dose necessary to raise it to 5 pg/ml was about one-tenth of that routinely prescribed in conventional medicine.

Postmenopausal women and oestrogen

Oestrogen levels decline at menopause, but not to zero. Oestradiol falls generally to about 15% of premenopausal levels, and oestrone falls only to 40 to 50% of premenopausal levels. Androstenedione, a hormone made in the ovary long after menopause, is converted in body fat into oestrone, which is partially converted in the gut and liver into oestradiol. Therefore, the question becomes: Is this oestrogen sufficient for normal bodily functions excluding pregnancy? That is, did Mother Nature intend that women should become estrogen deficient after menopause? I think not. *Oestrogen deficiency at menopause is a myth created by drug companies to justify selling supplemental oestrogen.*

It should be obvious that postmenopausal women do not need oestrogen levels so high that the endometrium is stimulated as much as it would be in preparing every month for pregnancy (i.e. premenopausal levels), but that is what is currently prescribed.

Use symptoms as a guide

Blood or saliva tests can measure your oestrogen levels, but symptoms alone can be a reliable indicator of oestrogen excess or deficiency. The symptoms of oestrogen deficiency are persistent vaginal dryness or vaginal mucosal atrophy (thinning), or persistent hot flushes despite adequate progesterone treatment. Oestrogen deficiency can also cause urinary tract problems. Postmenopausal women with these symptoms might benefit from small doses of oestrogen as a supplement. (See 'Oestrogen: which one and how much?' below for dosage information.)

The most common excess oestrogen symptoms are weight gain, water retention, breast swelling and lumpiness, headaches, hypertension, insomnia and anxiety.

Premenopausal women don't need oestrogen

Conventional medicine has long held that oestrogen production declines during premenopausal years. This is not true. Dr. Jerilyn C. Prior[9] thoroughly reviewed all pertinent references from 1990 to the present and found no evidence that oestrogen levels fall before menopause. All evidence indicates that overall oestrogen production remains at normal premenopausal levels,

It has also been assumed that premenopausal hot flushes are caused by oestrogen deficiency. If oestrogen levels are normal, what causes the hot flushes? It is fluctuating hormones against a background of progesterone deficiency. Remember, women begin to have non-ovulating menstrual cycles in their mid-thirties. Any month that you don't ovulate, you don't make any progesterone (although you will still have a menstrual period). Without progesterone you can't maintain good oestrogen receptor sensitivity, so even when there's plenty of oestrogen available, your cells can't use it as effectively.

Thus, treating the underlying progesterone deficiency first to reduce the overall hormone fluctuations allows you to take advantage of the oestrogen you have.

Oestrogen for hot flushes, heart disease and osteoporosis?

Even for women who have reached menopause, progesterone supplementation alone usually relieves hot flushes. As Dr. Helene Leonetti reports[10] from her ongoing study of osteoporosis treatment in recently menopausal women, the majority experienced excellent relief of hot flushes using progesterone cream alone.

Some argue that oestrogen provides protection against coronary heart disease, but we still don't have one good study proving this, because they have all been done either in combination with progestins (i.e. Provera), or with Premarin, which contains pregnant horse urine that has hundreds of active ingredients besides oestrogen, including progesterone and other steroid hormones.

A recent study of oestrogen and heart disease reported in the *Journal of the American Medical Association*[11] looked at prevention of coronary heart disease in postmenopausal women (average age 66.7 years). After an average follow up of 4 to 5 years, no difference in overall heart disease was observed relative to HRT using Premarin and Provera.

Some women lose bone very rapidly right around menopause. The decline of oestrogen combined with low progesterone may be more than the body can keep up with for a few years, even with supplemental progesterone. Most women regain bone balance and maintain good bone density within a few years after menopause, especially if they use progesterone cream. However, a small percentage of women with low oestrogen and oestrogen deficiency symptoms combined with indications of osteoporosis will benefit from using a small amount of supplemental oestrogen with progesterone at this time of their life. These women are often petite, thin (with not enough body fat to make significant oestrogen), and have small bones.

Handle with care

Oestrogen is necessary to maintain progesterone receptors; it is necessary to maintain good brain function and healthy bones; and a true oestrogen deficiency may compromise the ability of blood vessels to relax and thus help protect against a heart attack. But a true oestrogen deficiency in the 1990s is rare because we live in a highly oestrogen-contaminated world (see my book, *What Your Doctor May Not Tell You About Menopause*). When oestrogen levels are too high the risk of cancer increases steeply; its protective value in heart disease is reversed as the risk of blood clots and fluid imbalances rises; and the brain benefits are lost. Oestrogens are indeed the angels of life and the angels of death. They should be used only when needed, with moderation and respect, and with a goal of overall hormone balance.

Oestrogen: which one and how much?

There are many ways to increase oestrogen levels in the body. Here are some suggestions, from simple dietary changes to actual oestrogen supplementation.

1 **Diet modification** with less starch and more phytooestrogens (plant-based oestrogens) may be all that's needed. Avoid all processed foods and include plenty of fresh organic veggies, seeds, legumes (the bean family) and fish.

2 **Stress management** may help. Stress can increase cortisol levels that blockade progesterone from its receptors, thus down regulating oestrogen receptors as well. Further, stress can alter the production of pituitary hormones and endogenous oestrogen.

3 **Women who exercise regularly** pass through menopause with fewer problems.

4 **Consult with a herbalist** to select herbs containing phytooestrogens. In this regard, a trial of Remifemin is a possibility.

5 **Use of 'natural' (human) oestrogens**, i.e., oestrone, oestradiol, and oestriol. Each of these hormones differs in certain aspects, but with all of them the goal is to find the smallest dose that relieves symptoms and/or creates the desired blood or saliva level.

If used transdermally (as a cream or patch), both oestrone and oestradiol are well absorbed but oestriol is not well absorbed.

Oestriol is safer in regard to cancer risk than oestradiol or oestrone and is the preferred oestrogen for vaginal use. I have found good results with twice weekly vaginal dosing for 25 days a month, always along with progesterone. (The progesterone does not need to be used vaginally.) Begin with half the usual prescribed dose.

Since oestriol is considerably less potent than the others, orally it requires 1 to 2 mg/day for 25 days/month.

Oestrone is more potent, so orally 0.3 mg/day for 25 days/month should be sufficient, and many of my patients have found 0.5 mg every other day to be effective.

Oestradiol is the most potent, and for an oral dose I recommend only 0.25 mg/day for 25 days/month.

A more thorough discussion of the oestrogen's effects on breast fibrocysts, breast cancer, as well as on bones and the prevention or treatment of osteoporosis, will be presented in chapters to follow.

9

Progesterone and pelvic disorders

THE HUMAN FEMALE PELVIS is a wonder to behold. Its tissues are sufficiently elastic and its bony arches sufficiently large for passage of babies
with heads already over 50% the size of an adult's. Vaginal tissue during fertile
years, and especially at parturition, is the best healing tissue of the body.
Vaginal mucus secretions are responsive to and facilitate sexual activity; protective against infection; and promote self-cleansing. The ova-forming ovaries are
placed in the most protected spot of the body. The vaginal passage is positioned
so as to promote face-to-face intercourse, a rarity among all species of
animals. The uterus, normally smaller than a fist, can accommodate a pregnancy larger than a basketball, retain muscle strength sufficient for successful
delivery contractions, and return to normal within 6 weeks after delivery.
Despite its proximity to the rectum and the possibility of coliform contamination (the dreaded E. coli), a healthy pelvis is remarkably resistant to
infection, in spite of a monthly discharge of bloody flow that might otherwise
be a culture medium *par excellence*.

Pelvic disorders do, of course, occur. Conditions such as vaginitis, urinary
tract infections, endometriosis, PID (pelvic inflammatory disease), ovarian
cysts, Mittelschmerz, uterine fibroid and menstrual cramps (dysmenorrhoea)
come to mind. The question to be asked is: are these to be expected because
of some error in Nature's plan or do these occur because of some preventable
cause? Let us take a closer look.

Vaginitis

Vaginitis occurs more often among women taking contraceptive pills. One
might argue that taking contraceptive pills implies more frequent sexual
activity and, therefore, such women are more exposed to infectious organisms. Perhaps so, but one could also argue that contraceptive pills prevent the
normal hormone-generated mucus from being produced to protect them.
Birth control pills work, after all, by suppressing normal hormones.

After menopause, vaginal dryness and atrophic mucosa predispose women to vaginal, urethral and urinary bladder infections. To treat the infectious agent (pathogenic bacteria or whatever) with antibiotics is only temporarily successful because the underlying real cause of the problem is loss of *host resistance* secondary to hormone deficiency. In this regard, oestrogen by vaginal application has historically been remarkably successful, with oestriol being the most effective. A recent controlled trial[1] of intravaginal oestriol in post-menopausal women with recurrent urinary tract infections found that oestriol significantly reduced the incidence of urinary infections compared to placebo (0.5 versus 5.9 episodes per year). In addition, oestriol treatment resulted in the re-emergence of friendly Lactobacilli and the near elimination of colon bacteria as well as the restoration of normal vaginal mucosa and a resumption of normal low pH (which inhibits the growth of many pathogens).

In my care of postmenopausal patients, there are those for whom oestrogens are contraindicated by reason of history of breast or uterine cancer and who are at risk of recurrent urinary tract and vaginal infections. I have been surprised to observe that those who opted for natural progesterone therapy have been remarkably free of these problems. Further, their previous vaginal dryness and mucosal atrophy return to normal conditions after 3-4 months of progesterone use. This suggests that natural progesterone also provides a direct benefit to vaginal and urethral tissues or may sensitize tissue receptors to the lowered levels of oestrogens still present in postmenopausal women.

An important, yet unrecognized, aspect of host resistance is secretory IgA, an immune globulin which activates one's immune defenses *prior* to actual cellular invasion of tissue by pathogenic organisms. Secretory IgA is present in the normal secretions of the healthy vagina. Though not yet validated by adequate research, it is tempting to advance the hypothesis that natural hormones stimulate not only the normal quantity of mucus but also the normal components of mucus, including such items as secretory IgA. Further, it is likely that this immune mechanism, like others, is facilitated by nutritional aspects, also.

Pelvic inflammatory disease (PID)

PID is a serious inflammation of the uterus and Fallopian tubes which can result in pelvic abscesses. Its treatment includes antibiotics and. possibly, surgery. Infectious agents include gonorrhoea, chlamydia, and, most often, coliform bacteria. The progress of this disease originates from colonization of the infectious pathogen first in the vagina and cervical tissues with ascending infection into the endometrium and out along the Fallopian tubes, at which point the inflammation is called salpingitis or pelvic inflammatory disease (PID). Prevention, therefore, must rely on (1) reducing the opportunity of vaginal contamination (i.e., vaginal hygiene) and (2) increasing one's resistance to opportunistic pathogens. In both of these tactics, vaginal mucus is an important factor. Normal vaginal mucus results from normal balance of natural hormones and potential nutritional factors such as vitamins betacarotene, E, C and B-6 and the minerals zinc and magnesium. It is unlikely that synthetic hormones (i.e,. contraceptive pills and postmenopausal supplements) provide the hormone balance or action necessary for the most effective vaginal mucus.

As already noted, oestriol is the oestrogen most beneficial to vaginal and cervical tissue, the sites that act as the first line of defense against pathogens. Oestriol is a product of oestrone metabolism. Contraceptive synthetic oestrogens, which inhibit the production of natural hormones, do not contain oestriol and are not metabolized to form oestriol. Similarly, progestins inhibit production of natural progesterone. After menopause, progesterone levels fall to near-zero and oestrone levels are also low. Thus, the protection against vaginal colonization by pathogens as offered by oestriol and progesterone is lost and the risk of pelvic infection rises when contraception pills are used and/or after menopause unless natural hormones are used in supplementation.

Ovarian cysts and mittelschmerz

Ovarian cysts are products of failed or disordered ovulation. As described in Chapter 2, one or more ovarian follicles are developed monthly by the effects of follicle stimulating hormone (FSH). Luteinizing hormone (LH) promotes actual ovulation and the transformation of the follicle (after ovulation) into the corpus luteum which produces progesterone. In young women, during the early years of menstrual cycles, ovulation may coincide with a small amount of haemorrhage at the follicle site. This will cause abdominal pain, often with a slight fever, at the time of ovulation (in the middle days between periods) and is commonly called mittelschmerz (German for 'middle' and 'pain'). Treatment consists only of mild analgesics, reassurance, rest, and perhaps a warm pack. It is unlikely to recur and portends no future problems.

Later in life, usually after her mid-thirties, a woman may develop an ovarian cyst which may be asymptomatic or may cause variable pelvic pain.

Palpation may detect a smooth, tender mass at one ovary site or a cyst may be found by sonogram visualization. The cyst may simply collapse and disappear after a month or two; or it may persist and increase in size and discomfort during succeeding months. Such cysts are caused by a failed ovulation in which, for reasons presently unknown, the ovulation did not proceed to completion. With each succeeding month's surge of LH, the follicular site swells and stretches the surface membrane, causing pain and possible bleeding at the site. Some cysts may become as large as a golf ball or lemon before discovery. Treatment may require surgery during which the entire ovary may be lost.

An alternative treatment for ovarian cysts is natural progesterone (see pp122-3). Biofeedback mechanisms dictate that sufficient gonadal hormones inhibit hypothalamic and pituitary centres such that FSH and LH production are also inhibited. That is, in the usual circumstances, the successful response to FSH and LH hormones is the rise in progesterone from the corpus luteum. If sufficient natural progesterone is supplemented prior to ovulation, LH levels are inhibited and regular ovulation does not occur. This is the effect of contraception pills, for example. Similarly, the high oestriol and progesterone levels throughout pregnancy successfully inhibit ovarian activity for nine months. Therefore, adding natural progesterone from day 10 to day 26 of the cycle suppresses LH and its luteinizing effects. Thus, the ovarian cyst will not be stimulated and, in the passage of one or two such monthly cycles, will very likely regress and atrophy without further treatment.

Endometriosis

Endometriosis is a painful, devastating disease in which small islets of endometrial tissue somehow migrate into the muscular wall of the uterus, out along the Fallopian tubes, and even to the surface of the ovaries and the pelvic contents, including the nearby colon. When observed at surgery, these small islets appear as tiny chocolate-coloured blobs scattered here and there, some so small as to be nearly invisible to the unaided eye. Being endometrial tissue, they respond to the monthly surges of oestrogen and progesterone exactly like the endometrium within the uterus, i.e., they swell with blood during the month and then bleed at menses time, causing considerable pain starting shortly before menstruation and not subsiding until after menstruation. The small drops of blood trapped in the tissue in which the endometrial islets are embedded become chocolate coloured over time. When confined to the muscular wall of the uterus, the condition is called adenomyosis and can cause significant pain with menstruation, otherwise known as dysmenorrhoea.

The cause of this disorder is presently unknown. There is no mechanism known by which endometrial tissue could migrate throughout the pelvis as some cancers are able to. The hypothesis that scattered islets of endometrial tissue persist from embryonal time likewise is unproved. Further, the disorder appears to be of modern origin; it is difficult to imagine that such a painful disorder could have existed a century or two ago without some medical comment on it being made.

Some have hypothesized that it has something to do with the long time (and the many menses) between menarche and the first pregnancy. Until this century, women in the northern hemisphere typically experienced only two or three years of menstruation before becoming pregnant, menarche being at about age 16 and first pregnancies at about age 18 or 19. Now, menarche is common at age 12 and pregnancy is often delayed until after the mid-twenties. It has been calculated that the number of menses between menarche and first pregnancy was typically less than 30, whereas, now, it customarily exceeds 150. The outward migration of endometrial cells may somehow result from such a long run of menstrual cycling in sexually active women without the hormonal 'rest' of pregnancy. Further study is obviously needed.

Medical treatment of this disorder has included low-dose synthetic oestrogen (to suppress endogenous oestrogens), high-dose synthetic progestins taken daily or as long-acting IM injections of synthetic progestins (to suppress menses), and analgesics, including codeine and narcotics, for pain. The results are generally unsuccessful. The favourite treatment for young women with mild endometriosis is to recommend pregnancy as soon as possible. This is often successful when the recommended treatment can be followed.

Surgical treatment attempts to resect all visible endometrial lesions. This is rarely successful. Almost invariably, it becomes necessary to ablate (remove or destroy) both ovaries, tubes, and the uterus, regardless of the patient's age. When confined to the uterus (adenomyosis), hysterectomy is usually recommended.

Doctors may prescribe the birth control pill to ease the symptoms, but it often does not work well. Moreover, the potent progestins in the pill not only blockade real progesterone from its receptors, but also stop the ovary from producing any progesterone at all. So it is useless to use real progesterone when taking birth control pills.

Natural progesterone offers a more benign alternative. In women with endometriosis, the goal is to increase progesterone levels to those found in women two months pregnant.

My treatment for endometriosis is based on the well-known fact that endometriosis usually subsides during pregnancy. Unfortunately the symptoms often recur some time after delivery. The underlying endometriosis hypothesis is that oestrogen dominance stimulates proliferation of blood-rich tissue in the endometrium and in the endometriosis islets. At menstruation, the blood in these islets has nowhere to go and causes inflammation and severe pain in the various tissues where the islets are.

Progesterone stops the oestrogen-driven proliferative phase. By creating a pseudo-pregnant state from day 8 or 9 until day 26 of the menstrual cycle, this monthly proliferation of bloody tissue in the endometriosis islets is reduced. Over time, one's natural healing process will heal the endometriosis islets. Most patients find reduction of pain in three to four months, and continued relief as time goes by.

When endometriosis pains have subsided, the dose can be reduced gradually to find the level that keeps the pains away. After menopause, when oestrogen levels decline, the dose of progesterone can be reduced even further.

It is a mystery to me why synthetic progestins are recommended when the natural progesterone is available, cheaper, and safer.

Doses to use for endometriosis

The pseudo-pregnant state (from day 8 or 9 until day 26) is obtained by using about 40 to 50 mg of progesterone daily, applied topically in divided doses twice a day, usually at bedtime and in the morning.

Later, when pain symptoms have subsided considerably, the dose can be reduced to about 20 to 30 mg/day.

After menopause, the typical dose is about 15 mg/day for 25 to 26 days of the month.

Uterine fibroid tumour

Otherwise known as myoma of the uterus, fibroids are the most common neoplasm of the female genital tract. They are discrete, round, firm, benign lumps of the muscular wall of the uterus, composed of smooth muscle and connective tissue, and are rarely solitary. Usually as small as an egg, they grow gradually to orange or grapefruit size commonly. The largest fibroid on record weighed over a hundred pounds. They often cause or are coincidental with heavier periods (hypermenorrhoea), irregular bleeding (metrorrhagia), and/or painful periods (dysmenorrhoea). Due to their mass, they may cause a cystocele (dropped uterus) later in life when pelvic floor supports weaken, leading to stress urinary incontinence. After menopause, they routinely atrophy.

Contemporary medical treatment usually is surgical. Some particularly skillful surgeons are adept at excising only the myoma, leaving the uterus intact. Generally, however, hysterectomy is performed.

Here again, natural progesterone offers a better alternative. Fibroid tumours, like breast fibrocysts, are a product of oestrogen dominance. Oestrogen stimulates their growth and lack of oestrogen causes them to atrophy. Oestrogen dominance is a much greater problem than recognized by contemporary medicine. Many women in their thirties begin to have anovulatory cycles. As they approach the decade before menopause, they are producing much less progesterone than expected but still producing normal (or more) oestrogen. They retain water and salt, breasts swell and become fibrocystic, they gain weight (especially around the hips and torso), become depressed and lose libido, their bones suffer mineral loss, and they develop fibroids. All are signs of oestrogen dominance, i.e. relative progesterone deficiency.

When sufficient natural progesterone is replaced (see p123), fibroid tumours no longer grow in size (generally they decrease in size) and can be kept from growing until menopause after which they will atrophy. This is the effect of reversing oestrogen dominance. Anovulatory periods can be verified by checking serum progesterone levels the week following supposed ovulation. A low reading indicates lack of ovulation and the need to supplement with natural progesterone. The cause of anovulation is uncertain but probably attests to premature depletion of ovarian follicles secondary to environmental toxins and nutritional deficiencies common in the US today.

Endometrial carcinoma

This pelvic disorder is another example of oestrogen dominance. Unopposed oestrogen is the only known aetiology of endometrial carcinoma. Both natural progesterone and the synthetic progestins will protect a woman from this malady. This important topic will be discussed more thoroughly in Chapter 12.

Summary

The monthly rise and fall of natural oestrogen(s) and progesterone not only prepares the woman for procreation in the sense of ova production but also disposes the woman to be healthy. Many of the female pelvic complaints arise from an imbalance of her hormones. This imbalance is most often a deficiency of natural progesterone.

There are many factors that bring this about: nutritional deficiencies, stress, environmental xenooestrogens, toxins, follicular depletion, and, of course, the hormonal imbalance induced by contraception pills composed of synthetic hormones. Though this book is not designed to include full consideration of all these factors, it is important that they be acknowledged.

The major point to be made is that progesterone deficiency and oestrogen dominance can be recognized and handily treated by supplementation of natural progesterone, especially when combined with an approach that considers the multi-factorial heterogenicity of the underlying causes. Once that concept is grasped, a wide spectrum of female disorders now subject to invasive and traumatic procedures can be better treated with addition of natural progesterone.

10

Progesterone and PMS

PREMENSTRUAL SYNDROME (PMS) refers to a rather broad set of symptoms including several or all of the following; bloating, weight gain, headache, back aches, irritability, depression, breast swelling or tenderness, loss of libido, and fatigue; and that they occur consistently a week or ten days before menses and routinely relent with or shortly after menses. Symptoms are variable in intensity but often impact adversely on the patients' work capability and interpersonal relationships. Patients often report a 'tidal wave' of symptoms at their onset and dread the approach of each premenstrual time of the month. Because of the consistent premenstrual timing, a correlation with hormonal balance (imbalance?) is strongly suspected. Other hypotheses include emotional stress, nutritional factors, and genetic components.

Treatment of PMS has, in the past, included diuretics, tranquillizers, dietary changes, aerobic exercise, psychiatric counselling, thyroid supplements, herbs, acupuncture, and vitamin and mineral supplements. While each may provide some symptomatic improvement, it is clear that proper treatment still eludes discovery. A number of self-help organizations and newsletters have sprung up among victims of this disorder.

If one compares the symptoms of PMS with the side effects of oestrogen (see Chapters 7 and 8), the similarity is striking. A decade or so ago, after reading of the work of Dr. Katherine Dalton in London who defined the syndrome and found success using high-dose progesterone administered as rectal suppositories, I decided to add natural progesterone transdermally in my treatment of patients with PMS. The results were most impressive. The majority (but not all) of such patients reported remarkable improvement in their symptom-complex, including the elimination of their premenstrual water retention and weight gain. Since most of the symptoms are subjective, the objective finding of absence of premenstrual weight gain is of particular importance in verifying the benefits of natural progesterone in the treatment of PMS. Further, it helps to clarify and substantiate the hormone aetiology hypothesis.

As described in previous chapters, oestrogen is the dominant gonadal hormone during the first week after the menses. With ovulation, progesterone levels rise to assume dominance during the two weeks preceding menstruation. Progesterone blocks many of oestrogen's potential side effects. A surplus of oestrogen or a deficiency of progesterone during these two weeks allows an abnormal month-long exposure to oestrogen dominance, setting the stage for the symptoms of oestrogen side effects. The validity of this hypothesis can be checked by measuring serum progesterone levels during days 18-25 of the cycle. Low progesterone levels undoubtedly effect regulatory hypothalamic centres resulting in hyperactivity of these centres as well as increased production of FSH and LH gonadotropins. These, also, may play a role in the complex symptomatology of PMS. However, simple correction of the progesterone deficiency will restore normal biofeedback and normal pituitary function.

An important caveat should be inserted at this point. The word 'syndrome' refers to symptom complex, a set of symptoms that appear to occur together, and infers no specific aetiology (or that the aetiology is unknown). It is entirely possible that a number of the symptoms in the PMS complex may derive from causes other than relative progesterone deficiency. Hypothyroidism, for example, may present as fatigue, headaches, loss of libido, etc., and thus simulate PMS. Conversely, oestrogen dominance impairs the thyroid hormone activity and will simulate hypothyroidism. Differentiation of the two is possible by testing serum thyroid levels (T-3 and T-4) and thyroid stimulating hormone (TSH). Normal T-3 and T-4 levels with elevated TSH suggests impaired thyroid hormone activity rather than a true deficiency of thyroid hormone production. Similarly, persons with reactive hypoglycaemia often experience symptoms similar to PMS and will benefit from dietary adjustments. However, it should be known that oestrogen predisposes one to blood sugar imbalance whereas progesterone enhances blood sugar control. Further, there is no reason to suppose that the syndrome may not involve multiple factors working together. Thus, it is likely that, while relative progesterone deficiency may be the major factor in the majority of PMS cases, there may also be other factors that deserve attention, especially in those cases that do not find complete relief with progesterone treatment.

Deeper yet is the question — why would a relatively young (early or mid-thirties) woman experience progesterone deficiency? Is PMS a 'normal' occurrence among women or is it secondary to other factors peculiar to our culture or some other circumstance? Anthropologists tell us of cultures where the condition is unknown and essentially non-existent. Nutritional demands of menstrual cycling must be met for normal function. Thus, nutritional deficiencies common to our industrialized society probably play a role. Xenooestrogens, recently identified, may also play a role in hormone imbalance. Stress is a well known cause of menstrual irregularity. The advent of PMS after a time of contraception pill use is not uncommon, suggesting that synthetic hormone use and the prevention of normal ovulation may leave one's ovaries less able to function normally. All these, and others, must be considered in understanding and treating PMS. Recognizing this, the problem of normalizing hormone balance remains a key factor in proper treatment.

Dr. Joel T. Hargrove of Vanderbilt University Medical Centre has published results indicating a 90% success rate in treating PMS with oral doses of natural progesterone.[1] This correlates well with my experience in treating PMS with transdermal natural progesterone. The only difference is that his patients required about 5-8 times the daily dose to obtain the same effects as are needed when using progesterone transdermally. Oral progesterone is absorbed from the gut and transferred via the portal vein to the liver where much is metabolized and conjugated by glucuronic acid for excretion in the bile. This first pass liver loss reduces the effectiveness of oral progesterone by about 80%; whereas progesterone, like oestrogen and testosterone, is well absorbed transdermally. (See Chapter 12.)

Because other factors may work to create symptoms fitting the PMS complex, care of those patients who do not find relief from natural progesterone requires that these other factors (such as nutrition, stress, and environmental) must also be taken into account.

Summary
Though not completely understood, PMS most commonly represents an individual reaction to oestrogen dominance secondary to relative progesterone deficiency. Appropriate treatment requires correction of this hormone imbalance and the most effective technique, at present, for achieving this is supplemental natural progesterone.

For further suggestions on dosage, see pp121-122.

11

Progesterone and osteoporosis

OSTEOPOROSIS IS A MULTI-FACTORIAL SKELETAL DISORDER of progressive bone mass loss and demineralization causing an increased risk of fracture. Postmenopausal osteoporosis refers to the acceleration of this disorder in women after menopause. It is the most common metabolic bone disorder in the US, afflicting the great majority of postmenopausal women, annually causing over 1.3 million fractures at an estimated cost of over $10 billion. The personal cost in quality and quantity of life is incalculable. The most common osteoporotic fractures are of the vertebra, distal forearm, proximal femur (hip), proximal humerus (shoulder) and ribs, with hip fracture the most costly and most likely to be disabling. It occurs earlier and with greater severity in white women of northern European extraction who are relatively thin, and is more common among those who smoke cigarettes, are under-exercised, deficient in vitamin D, calcium, or magnesium, and in those whose diet is meat based rather than vegetable and wholegrain based. Also, alcoholism is a potent risk factor. Further, a genetic component is likely.

Bone mass in women is highest during their early or mid-thirties after which there occurs a gradual decline until menopause when the loss rate accelerates for 3-5 years and then typically continues at the rate of 1-1.5% per year. The menopausal acceleration of bone loss, first noted by F. Albright, P. H. Smith, and A. M. Richardson in 1941,[1] suggested that the decline in sex hormones is a causative factor. In the mid-1970s, oestrogen replacement after oophorectomy was found to lessen the loss of bone mass when compared to untreated oophorectomized control patients.[2,3] Oestrogen's role in osteoporosis was further supported by epidemiologic studies that demonstrated women treated with oestrogen sustained fewer fractures than did untreated women.[4-8] As Barzel[9] and others have pointed out, however, the earlier studies suffer from a number of defects including inadequate sample size, insufficient duration, and lack of precise bone density measurement technology, relying instead on fracture incidence end points or radiographic morphometry. In addition, these studies tended to include a disproportionate number of otherwise healthy women who had undergone oophorectomy or had experienced hot flushes. It is now generally agreed, however, that oestrogen therapy retards osteoporosis progression but does not truly prevent or reverse it.

During this same time period, it became evident that oestrogen replacement therapy was not without risk. Oestrogen unopposed by progesterone was found to cause salt and water retention, increase blood clotting, promote fat synthesis, oppose thyroxin, promote uterine fibroids, promote mastadynia and breast fibrocysts, increase risk of cholelithiasis, cholecystitis, and liver dysfunction, and, more ominously, increase the risk of endometrial cancer, pituitary prolactinoma, and , probably, breast cancer. Further, it was found that the bone benefits of oestrogen replacement after menopause wanes after 3-5 years. Thus, Barzel, after reviewing 31 oestrogen osteoporosis treatment studies (1972-1987), concluded that 'in post-menopausal women with established osteoporosis, oestrogen therapy may not be of significant benefit and may be associated with a high rate of unacceptable side effects and complications.'[9]

Contemporary medicine strangely persists in the single-minded belief that oestrogen is the mainstay of osteoporosis treatment for women. This is exceedingly odd because even the most authoritative medical textbooks do not support it, as the following examples illustrate.

- *Cecil's Textbook of Medicine*, 18th edition, 1988: 'Oestrogen is more effective than calcium but has significant side effects.' Recall that, above an essential minimum, additional calcium intake has little or no effect on osteoporosis.

- *Harrison's Principles of Internal Medicine*, 12th edition, 1991: 'Oestrogens may decrease the rate of bone resorption, but bone formation usually does not increase and eventually decreases' and 'oestrogens retard bone loss ... although restoration of bone mass is minimal', meaning inconsequential.

- *Scientific American's* updated *Medicine* text, 1991: 'Oestrogens decrease bone resorption' but 'associated with the decrease in bone resorption is a decrease in bone formation. Therefore, oestrogens should *not* be expected to increase bone mass.' (Emphasis added.) The authors also discuss oestrogen side effects including the risk of endometrial cancer which 'is increased six-fold in women who receive oestrogen therapy for up to five years; the risk is increased 15-fold in long-term users.'

If one pursues the supporting references for these lukewarm endorsements of oestrogen replacement therapy, the evidence favouring oestrogen's putative bone benefits becomes even more clouded. *None* of the strictly oestrogen studies showed any increase of bone mass. The modest increase of bone mass reported by Claus Christiansen, et al.[10] occurred in postmenopausal women given oestrogen *and* a progestin (noresthisterone acetate). From the data presented, there is no way to determine which, if either, was the responsible agent.

It should be noted that, since the mid-1970s when the oestrogen/endometrial cancer link was noted, all studies of hormone supplementation in postmenopausal women for osteoporosis have included a progestin along with the oestrogen. The potential confounding effect of progestins was simply never considered.

Moreover, the pharmaceutical industry viewed the potential osteoporosis market as a magnificent opportunity to sell their patent medicine hormones. Doctors were treated to massive advertising campaigns via journal advertisements, promotional symposia disguised as 'continuing medical education' (i.e., CME, a requirement for physicians these days) with appropriate credits, personal visits by drug salesmen bringing boxes of free samples, and medical articles of studies spawned by generous grants from the industry, all touting the putative bone benefit of oestrogen and the protective effect (against endometrial cancer) of progestins. In the past few years, Prior et al have provided reliable evidence that osteoporotic bone loss occurs in women with progesterone deficiency despite adequate oestrogen levels.[11] Yet, physicians continue to be taught that 'oestrogen is the single most potent factor in prevention of bone loss'.[12] The strength of the oestrogen-fixed mindset represents a victory of advertising over science.

A little bone physiology

Bones are living tissue and, unlike teeth, they can grow as the body grows, mend when broken, and continually renew themselves throughout life. Bone can be thought of as mineralised cartilage. The skeleton begins developing early in foetal life, and grows under the influence of pituitary growth hormone until puberty when the gonadal (sex) hormones come into play. Bone is largely composed of *osteoid*, a non-cellular collagenous matrix which becomes mineralized for greater strength. In addition to supporting our weight, muscles attached to bone account for their movement and impose the force of torsion when we lift heavy objects or move against resistance. Thus, bones are designed for compression strength and tensile strength. Animals, such as sharks, which are buoyant in water but have great muscle strength for swimming, have skeletons which do not require being mineralized. Other animals, e.g., jellyfish, also buoyant and lacking true muscles, have no skeleton at all.

Bone forming cells (osteocytes) differentiate into osteoclast and osteoblast varieties. Osteoclast cells continually travel through bone tissue looking for older bone previously mineralized and in need of renewal. Osteoclasts *resorb* (dissolve away) such bone leaving tiny unfilled spaces (lacunae) behind. Osteoblasts then move into these spaces and produce new bone. This astounding process of continual resorption (by osteoclasts) and new bone formation (by osteoblasts), called *remodelling,* is the mechanism for the remarkable repair abilities and the continuing strength of our bones.

At any stage in life, one's bone status is a product of the balance between these two functions of bone resorption and new bone formation. If the two processes are in balance, bone mass and bone strength remain constant. During the years of our major skeletal growth, osteoblast-mediated new bone formation dominates. During one's post-pubertal years, the processes are usually balanced. *Osteoporosis* is bone mass loss as the result of osteoclast dominance, i.e., more osteoclast-mediated bone resorption than osteoblast-mediated new bone formation. Decreased bone mass may also result from deficiency of a variety of other essential factors, e.g., calcium, vitamin D, etc. When this occurs it is variously referred to as rickets, osteomalacia, or the more generic, *osteopenia.*

The rate at which bone tissues renew themselves, called turnover rate, is quite remarkable. Dense bone (termed *cortical* bone) of the shafts of long bones is tightly cast in long cylindrical strands surrounding minute tubular channels (the *canaliculi*) for passage of nutrient vessels and osteocytes. The density and structure of cortical bone provide great tensile strength. The turnover time for 100% renewal is about 10-12 years. Other less dense bone, (termed *trabecular* [meaning 'little beams'] bone) needing only compression strength, is constructed as an open meshwork of little struts, and is found mostly at the ends of long bones, in the heel bone, and in vertebral bones. The 100% turnover time for these bones is about 4-5 years. Thus, osteoporosis will show itself earlier in trabecular bone than in cortical bone. Likewise, the progression of (or the recovery from) osteoporosis will be revealed earlier in trabecular bone. This, as will become evident, is of clinical significance.

Getting diagnosis and treatment in perspective

At a talk I gave last year, a woman named Sandy asked a question I hear daily.

'I'm not even menopausal,' she said, 'and yet I tested as having low bone mineral density. My doctor says this is very serious and wants me to start taking Fosamax and oestrogen right away. I've heard terrible things about Fosamax from friends, and my aunt has breast cancer so I'm afraid of oestrogen. What should I do?'

Sandy didn't have oestrogen deficiency symptoms such as hot flushes or night sweats, but she did have some oestrogen dominance symptoms (see Chapters 7 and 8), was overweight, and was clearly approaching menopause. She was also very petite and didn't get much exercise. When BMD is tested, petite bones result in lower readings than larger bones of the same true density (see page 74). Also, good exercise helps build stronger bones. Since she is still having menstrual periods, there is no reason to add oestrogen. This would be a good time to check her serum or saliva progesterone level and, if low, she could add physiologic doses of progesterone during the luteal phase (last two weeks) of her menstrual cycle.

I recommended she avoid Fosamax because it can have serious side effects. Another little-told fact is that the drug has a 10-15 year half-life in the body. Because it is chemically bound to protein, it becomes incorporated into the bone itself and blocks bone resorption, which is the process by which old, weak bone is removed to make room for new bone. *Your goal is not to block bone resorption, it's to balance bone resorption and bone-building.*

Although I am giving you a lot of information about bones and bone density, the bottom line is that you do not need to panic, or be pressured or frightened into taking drugs, if you have a low bone density reading. Bone density can be an important indicator of bone health and the progress of osteoporosis treatment, but it has to be interpreted correctly.

Reducing fracture risk takes more than good bone density

The other reason I don't want you to panic or be pressured is that there are many effective, practical, and safe steps you can take to rapidly increase your bone density. These are covered in detail in Chapter 12 of my book, *What Your Doctor May Not Tell You About Menopause*.

The latest research published since I wrote that book is even more encouraging. Just adding soy to your diet a few times a week (don't overdo it) can raise your bone density by as much as 6%. Weight-bearing exercise alone can stop the bone loss process in its tracks and add 1-2%of bone mass a year.

Does a low BMD mean a hip fracture?

Contrary to what you'd expect, BMD has not been found to be a good predictor of future fractures. This was clearly shown in a nine-year study done in France, of 7,575 women aged 75 or older, with no history of hip fracture. The results show that poor balance, reduced vision, lack of muscle strength and lack of coordination were as important as bone density in predicting hip fractures.[13]

This means that even if your bone density is good, you need the additional protection of staying strong and coordinated, and if you're strong and coordinated your risk of fracture will be reduced even if your bone density is low.

A similar study done in the U.S. and published in the *New England Journal of Medicine* (NEJM) in 1995 had very similar results,[14] and the 1998 European Congress on Osteoporosis came to similar conclusions.

Other important causes of fractures in women include taking drugs that cause dizziness, such as sleeping pills and drugs that lower blood pressure, and taking drugs that deplete bone, such as cortisone.

Keep this in mind

Osteoporosis is a multi-faceted metabolic disease. Proper hormone balance is important, of course, but other factors are also important. Again, both are described in detail in *What Your Doctor May Not Tell You About Menopause*. They include exercise, nutrition, certain specific vitamins and minerals, sufficient stomach acid, and even stress management (stress produces cortisol, which blocks progesterone from its receptors). If a woman's bones do not improve with supplemental progesterone and oestrogen, it is usually an indication that one or more of the other osteoporosis factors needs to be attended to. Consulting with a knowledgeable health care professional will help you find the factors that, when corrected, will help restore good bones.

What your doctor may not know about bone density measurement

It's a useful tool, but not a gold standard

Ronnie, a petite, 105-pound, 45-year-old woman wrote to me in alarm after her doctor told her she had osteoporosis. Her lumbar (BMD) was low, and her doctor wanted her to take Fosamax. I assured her that, for her petite size, her BMD was just fine and she could stick to her good diet and plenty of exercise.

Conversely, Peggy, a rather large woman with a BMD in the 'normal' range, asked why she had several compression fractures on her spine. She had been told she did not have osteoporosis. I explained that, for her size, her bone BMD should be higher, and that she needed osteoporosis treatment.

This type of confusion is created by the limitations of the tests themselves. Testing techniques include dual-energy X-ray absorptiometry (DEXA), dual photon absorptiometry (DPA), quantified CT scan (QCT) and more recently, quantitative ultrasound (QUS) or broadband ultrasound attenuation (BUA) which are still experimental. Each technique measures slightly different bone characteristics and provides slightly different results. *This means that if you want to compare your BMD results over time (serial testing), you should use the same technique each time.*

Let's talk about DEXA and DPA, the most common techniques. An X-ray or photon (light) beam is directed at a body site such as the hip or lumbar spine, and the energy of the beam as it exits the body is measured. As the beam passes through the body, some of it is deflected or absorbed by striking minerals. Only the particles that don't hit a mineral will pass through the tissue and can be measured as they exit. The more minerals in the path of the beam, the greater the loss of beam energy. From this drop in beam energy, a computer calculates the mass of bone minerals encountered by the beam in its passage through the body. This is then reported as bone mineral density (BMD).

What does bone density really mean?

The use of the word 'density' in BMD creates some confusion, because you would think that two women with the same amount of minerals in, say, a postage stamp-sized section of bone would have the same BMD. But this is not true because BMD levels vary depending on the size of a woman's bones, as well as on the concentration of minerals in that bone. Because a larger person generally has larger bones than a smaller person does, the energy beam going through a large person's bones will encounter more minerals than it would if it traversed a smaller person's smaller bones of the same density. This means that even if the true densities of both bones are identical, the result of DEXA or DPA tests will indicate a higher 'density' in the larger person's larger bones.

Thus there are no BMD levels that are 'high', 'low' or 'normal' for everyone: what is normal for one woman may be low or high for another, and what is low for another woman may be perfectly fine for a third.

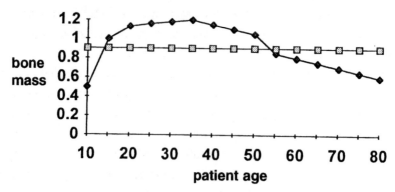

Figure 4. Bone mass (gms/cm²) relative to a woman's age. Schematic graph of bone mass relative to age, with menopause at age 50. Bone mass below horizontal line represents level of increased fracture risk. Note the more rapid decrease in bone mass during the five years after menopause. Note also that bone mass loss starts a number of years before actual menopause.

Use BMD measure for treatment

Despite the shortcomings of BMD testing, it is still valuable as an index of the effectiveness of any osteoporosis therapy you may be receiving: in other words you can compare your own readings for progress.

BMD is not accurate, however in two cases. Anti-resorptive drugs such as the bisphosphonates (oetidronate/Didronel and alendronate/Fosamax) inhibit resorption of old bone, leading to a rise in BMD even though the skeleton will be composed of older bone of less tensile strength. Also, elevated fluoride levels in the body, usually due to fluoridated water, result in bone which is denser but of poorer quality, but which will also yield a higher BMD reading (see 'Bone collagen and fluoride' below).

Excluding these two exceptions, a rise in BMD while on osteoporosis therapy is a sign of bone improvement.

This is why I want you to use BMD as a tool to analyse your bone health, but I don't want you to panic at a low reading. It may or may not be entirely accurate, it isn't necessarily predictive of a fracture, and there's plenty you can do to improve your bone density without resorting to Fosamax.

Bone collagen and fluoride

Bone mineral density (BMD) is not the sole factor in bone strength. Bone collagen (the non-mineralized matrix of bone) is also important. Poor bone collagen reduces bone strength, but is not measured by BMD. Poor bone collagen is the result of poor nutrition, lack of exercise, and total fluoride intake.

Fluoride is particularly toxic to collagen production, affecting not only the quantity but also the quality of the collagen. In the presence of fluoride, the micro-architecture of collagen fibres is disordered, leading to a lack of tensile strength. After thirty-plus years of studying the effects of fluoride on humans, I believe that this is the main cause of the increased incidence of hip fracture in communities with fluoridated water. Collagen fragmentation due to fluoride also leads to the inflammation and eventual destruction of cartilage, and the loss of 'cushioning' effect in the event of falls.

The progesterone hypothesis

As noted above, osteoporosis in women typically starts in their mid-thirties, often fifteen years before menopause, with a bone loss rate of about 1% per year. With menopause, bone loss accelerates to 3-5% per year for 5 years or so, after which bone loss continues at the rate of about 1.5% per year. If the oestrogen hypothesis of osteoporosis were true, there would be no reason for the premenopausal bone mass loss when oestrogen levels remain high. Clearly, there is something wrong with the oestrogen hypothesis. Perhaps the more important hormone is progesterone. It is during these years prior to menopause that *progesterone* levels fall, due to anovulatory periods.

The accelerated loss of bone as a consequence of menopause suggests the additional effect of oestrogen loss. Recall, however, that this stage of accelerated loss lasts for only 4-5 years and then resumes the more typical loss rate of 1-1.5% per year,[15] suggesting that the oestrogen effect is subject to adaptive adjustment by bone cells.

Present evidence suggests that oestrogen's actions regarding bone are related solely to osteoclast mediation of bone resorption. Manolagas et al reported[16] that the *lack* of oestrogen stimulates production of interleukin-6 which stimulates growth of osteoclasts, thus increasing bone resorption. There is no convincing evidence that oestrogen stimulates new bone formation. This effect of oestrogen lack causing increased osteoclast-mediated bone resorption is most noticeable in the 5 years immediately following menopause. After that period, continued use of oestrogen is relatively ineffective, with bone loss proceeding at the same rate as in those not on oestrogen.[15]

On the other hand, Prior has presented the evidence[17] that progesterone does have receptors in osteoblasts and is more likely, therefore, to effect new bone formation. Further, several small studies[18-21] have shown modest bone benefit (though less than that from natural progesterone) from use of synthetic progestins. From the available evidence, several deductions can be made.

- Oestrogen retards osteoclast-mediated bone resorption.
- Natural progesterone stimulates osteoblast-mediated new bone formation.
- Some progestins may also stimulate new bone formation to a lesser degree.

Since it is clear that (1) oestrogen can retard but not reverse osteoporosis, and (2) oestrogen can not protect against osteoporosis when progesterone is absent, the addition of natural progesterone should be beneficial in preventing or treating postmenopausal osteoporosis. Further, since some oestrogen is produced endogenously in postmenopausal women, it is possible that progesterone alone is sufficient to prevent and/or reverse osteoporosis. This is, in fact, what occurs. I have, since 1982, treated postmenopausal osteoporosis with transdermal natural progesterone cream included in a programme of diet, mineral and vitamin supplements, and modest exercise, and demonstrated true reversal of osteoporosis even in patients who did not use oestrogen supplements.[22-24]

Figure 5 illustrates the typical difference in bone mineral density (BMD) changes over a 3-year period between a group of 63 patients using progesterone supplementation, the typical effect of oestrogen treatment, and natural course of untreated controls.

In this graph, it can be seen that the untreated postmenopausal patient with osteoporosis will lose 1.5 % bone mass per year; that oestrogen supplementation will tend to maintain bone mass; but only the addition of natural progesterone will increase bone mass, thus reversing the osteoporotic process.

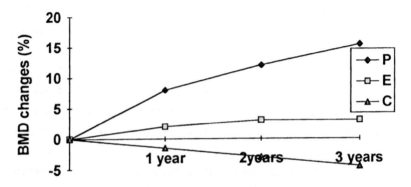

Figure 5. Typical 3-year changes in bone marrow density using progesterone (P), oestrogen (E), and controls (C) (i.e. without hormone therapy).

A minority of the patients using transdermal natural progesterone were also given low-dose oestrogen for treatment of vaginal dryness while the majority used no oestrogen. Approximately 40% of the progesterone-treated patients had been on oestrogen supplements prior to starting progesterone and most discontinued their oestrogen if not needed for vaginal dryness. Those with the lowest initial lumbar BMD readings showed the greatest response to progesterone. Also, a comparison of patients younger than 70 years of age with those over 70 showed no difference in their bone response to progesterone. Further, patients who are now well up in their eighties continue to enjoy strong bones without evident bone loss while continuing their use of natural progesterone. Age is not the cause of osteoporosis; poor nutrition, lack of exercise, and progesterone deficiency are the major factors.

Other osteoporosis factors

Effective treatment of postmenopausal osteoporosis requires regard of a number of factors known to influence bone building. It is likely that, in the future, even more will become known and additional strategies employed. Bone building should be considered as a chain of linked factors, each of which must be strong for the chain to be strong. Since calcium is the predominant mineral in bone building, it is helpful to follow the chain of events (see above) that facilitate its bone use from ingestion to incorporation into bone.

Each of these will be briefly considered in turn.

1. Calcium

The role of calcium in bone building is the most widely known. When other factors are properly taken care of, one's intake of calcium should be about 0.6-0.8 grams (600-800 mg) daily. Approximately 98-99% of body calcium is in taken up by bones where it is used (a) in bone mineralization, and (b) as a reservoir from which calcium can be taken to satisfy other homeostatic demands such as serum calcium levels, a process primarily facilitated by *parathyroid* hormone.

The source of all calcium is from Earth's soil and our primary edible source is plants (broad leaf vegetables especially) which incorporate calcium into their structure along with other minerals, vitamins, and energy-rich compounds which facilitates its absorption. Calcium, to be absorbed, requires *both* gastric HCl and vitamin D. Older people (usually over 70) often lack sufficient gastric acid for good absorption. This can be corrected, if and when it is detected, by HCl supplements taken with meals. The common perception,

	Facilitating factors
Ingested calcium	
↓	Gastric hydrochloric acid (HCl) and vitamin D
Absorbed calcium	
↓	Exercise, progesterone (stimulates osteoblasts),
↓	oestrogen (restrains osteoclasts), magnesium,
↓	micronutrients. Avoid excess protein, diuretics,
↓	antibiotics, fluoride and metabolic acidosis.
Bone incorporation	

sponsored by the dairy association, is that dairy products are the primary source of calcium. Missing from this amusing perception is the fact that well over 70% of the people on earth live in the equatorial zone (between the tropic of Cancer and the tropic of Capricorn), where food plants grow the year around and cows' milk is not used. These people have better bones than we in the more-northern, industrialized areas have. Also missing from the dairy perception is the fact that cows get the calcium for their bones and milk from plants they eat.

Other factors being equal, vegetarians uniformly have better mineralized bone than omnivores (that include meat in their diet). Meat is high in protein and the urinary excretion of protein waste products causes excessive loss of calcium, called a *negative calcium balance*. It is true that some people can adapt to high meat diets by ingesting and absorbing more calcium to balance this urinary calcium loss, but this strategy is unnecessary if one's diet is primarily vegetarian. In the US, contemporary medicine advocates 1200-1500 mg calcium per day (twice what is needed by vegetarians) for osteoporosis prevention.

Calcium incorporation into bone is a function of enzymes which require magnesium as a co-catalyst. If magnesium is deficient, calcium is less likely to become bone and more likely to appear as calcification of tendon insertion points, periarticular tissues, and joints, leading to tendonitis, bursitis, arthritis, and bone spurs. Good bone building thus requires not only calcium but adequate magnesium, of which our typical diet is deficient. (See 'Magnesium' below.)

If calcium supplementation is indicated, one should know that not all calcium supplements are equal. Calcium carbonate is the least expensive but is also the least well absorbed. This is relatively unimportant because higher doses can be easily used. Calcium citrate is more expensive but results in better calcium absorption when gastric HCl is low. Thus, it may be preferred for older patients.

2. Phosphorus

Phosphorus is the second most prevalent mineral in bones. Bone experts regard an ideal phosphorus/calcium intake ratio to be below 1.5:1. Excess phosphorus intake causes an imbalance of this ratio, leading to *decrease* in calcium absorption.

In bone formation, the proper ratio of phosphorus and calcium is important. Calcium and phosphates initially combine as amorphous tricalcium phosphate which is converted in a non-reversible hydrolysis process into crystalline hydroxyapatite, $[Ca_3(PO_4)_2]_3,- Ca(OH)_2$. If phosphorus is high, relative to calcium, osteoclasts increase in size, number and activity in response to parathyroid hormone (PTH), leading to enhanced osteoclast activity and bone resorption. This action is dependent on nearby osteoblasts which are the primary targets for PTH as osteoclasts contain no PTH receptors. PTH triggers osteoblasts to release local effectors (possibly interleukin 1 or a prostaglandin) which serve to stimulate osteoclasts to resorb bone. Thus, even though phosphorus is needed by bones, an excess of phosphorus, relative to calcium, can actually lead to bone loss. Since the typical US diet is, in fact, high in phosphorus, its supplementation is not indicated. 'Soda' drinks (artificially carbonated beverages previously called phospho-sodas) are high in phosphorus and low in calcium, as is red meat, and both should be restricted.

3. Magnesium

Magnesium, the third most prevalent mineral in bones, not only *increases* calcium absorption but facilitates its role in bone mineralization. Magnesium deficiency is common in the US, due to our food growing techniques, our food processing and our diet choices. This important mineral is normally abundant in nuts, seeds, grains, and vegetables of all sorts, the diet of our ancestors. Our grains, originally high in magnesium, are 'refined', a process which removes the outer fibrous coat along with its magnesium, zinc and other minerals. We eat more meat (low in magnesium) and dairy products (with a poor magnesium to calcium ratio). Our use of fertilizer that contains large amounts of potassium, a magnesium antagonist, results in foods lower in magnesium than ever before. Further, sugar and alcohol consumption both will increase urinary excretion of magnesium, leading to magnesium deficiency.

Interestingly, chocolate is high in magnesium. Chocolate craving is often a sign of magnesium deficiency and this craving will fade when magnesium intake is raised to adequate levels.

As described above, magnesium deficiency impairs utilization of calcium for bone building and results in calcium deposits in soft tissue rather than bone. In magnesium deficiency, calcium deficiency develops despite supposedly adequate supplementation. When adequate magnesium is supplied, calcium levels also rise, even without calcium supplementation. Thus, proper dietary choices and adequate magnesium supplementation are vital to healthy bones.

4. Other bone building minerals

Zinc is essential as a co-catalyst for enzymes which convert betacarotene to vitamin A within cells. The is especially important in building the collagen matrix of cartilage and bone. As with magnesium, zinc is one the minerals lost in the 'refining' of grain. As a result, the typical US diet is deficient in zinc and modest supplementation (15-30 mg/day) is recommended.

Manganese, boron, strontium, silicon and copper are also involved in building healthy bones. A diet of unprocessed foods is usually sufficient in providing these minerals.

5. Vitamin D

Vitamin D is essential for calcium and phosphorus transport from the intestine into the blood plasma; it causes re-absorption of calcium and phosphate from urine as it passes through renal tubules; and it facilitates mineralization of bones. Thus it is a key player in bone building. If vitamin D is deficient in young children, bones are incompletely mineralized and results in enlarged wrists, ankles and bowed legs, a condition named rickets. First described in 1650 by Professor Glisson of Cambridge, it was not until the early part of this century that rickets was learned to be limited to populations which lacked either fish oils or sufficient skin exposure to sunlight.[25] The missing factor came to be called vitamin D, being the fourth vitamin to be discovered (after A, B, and C). The same disease in adults is called osteomalacia (soft bones) or the more generic term, osteopenia (bone deficiency).

The synthesis of vitamin D in the skin follows a path from 7-dehydrocholesterol which, by the effect of ultraviolet light, undergoes scission (cutting, as with a scissors) of the B ring to form 'pre'-vitamin D_3 which is then modified to form vitamin D_3, or cholecalciferol, the natural vitamin D found in fish oils.

A second form of vitamin D can be obtained by irradiating ergosterol with ultraviolet light, creating vitamin D_2, or ergocalciferol, which differs only slightly in the structure of its side chain and is biologically identical to D_3.

In the forty years since its discovery, it has been found that vitamin D must undergo a further metabolic conversion to the active form, 1,25-dihydroxy-vitamin D_3. This involves one hydroxylation at the C-25 position (by the liver) and then another at the C-1 position (by the kidney).

In the manufacture of vitamin D_2, a plant sterol, ergosterol, is irradiated with ultraviolet light. In the skin, 7-dehydrocholesterol which is synthesized from cholesterol, is converted by ultraviolet light into vitamin D_3 (cholecalciferol). Biologically, the two are equivalent.

For reasons not yet known, the kidney produces both 1,25 $(OH)_2$ - D_3 and 24,25 $(OH)_2$ - D_3. In fact, plasma concentration of the latter (which has little or no calcium or bone building effect) is approximately 100 times that of the former, i.e. 1,25 $(OH)_2$ - vitamin D_3.

Rarely, a patient may have normal plasma levels of D_2 but deficient in 1,25 $(OH)_2$ - D_3, indicating a defect in the normal conversion of D_2. Patients whose blood tests confirm low levels of this metabolite despite normal D_2 need supplementation of 1,25 $(OH)_2$ - D_3 instead of the usual cholecalciferol.

Vitamin D deficiency is common during winter months (when more of the skin is covered by clothing) and is common among the elderly. Supplementation with 300-400 iu of vitamin D (cholecalciferol) is sufficient for most patients. High doses of vitamin D continued over a long period are *not* recommended due to the possibility of calcium deposition in soft tissues such as synovial membranes (leading to arthritis), the kidneys, the myocardium, the pancreas and the uterus.

6. Vitamin A

Vitamin A is important in the synthesis of connective tissue and the collagen matrix of cartilage and bone. It is normally produced intracellularly by metabolism of betacarotene, the vitamin A precursor found in yellow and deep green vegetables such as carrots, peppers, yams, sweet potatoes, string beans, leafy greens, melons (but not the Honeydew melon with its pale green interior), and many other vegetables and fruits. The metabolic conversion of betacarotene is inefficient if insufficient zinc is present to serve as an enzyme co-catalyst. The typical US diet is deficient in zinc, due primarily to the common use of refined grain. Thus, it is wise to recommend a supplement of betacarotene *and* zinc. Fish oil vitamin A may also be used but, being fat soluble, much of it is lost in the liver and excess vitamin A obtained in this fashion can be toxic to the liver and brain.

7. Vitamin C (ascorbic acid)

This vitamin is essential to the synthesis and repair of all collagen, including cartilage and the matrix of bone. Throughout the animal kingdom, vitamin C is synthesized by all but a very few species — the rind-eating bat in India, the Rhesus monkey, the guinea pig, the parakeet, and humans — at a daily rate of about 4 grams per 150 lbs of animal. Most of the non-vitamin C-producing animals choose (if free to do so) a diet which provides them with that amount of vitamin C. The typical US diet provides about 60 mg of vitamin C, or 1/70 of the animal standard. Generally, an adequate supplement of vitamin C should be not less than 2 grams per day.

8. Vitamin K

This valuable vitamin, necessary for normal blood clotting, is also a beneficial factor in bone building. Studies indicate vitamin K will reduce calcium excretion and will facilitate binding of osteocalcin (an important bone protein) to hydroxyapatite crystal. Fortunately for most of us, our colon bacteria synthesize sufficient quantities daily under normal circumstances. Prolonged use of broad-spectrum antibiotics, however, may reduce intestinal flora such that vitamin K production is deficient for us. Such patients may need supplemental vitamin K not only for maintaining normal blood clotting but also for its benefit to bone and the prevention of osteoporosis.

9. Vitamin B6 (pyridoxine)

Pyridoxal-5′-phosphate, the active form of vitamin B6, is a co-catalyst along with magnesium for a large number of enzymes. As such, it is a facilitator in the production of progesterone and reduces inflammatory reactions in connective tissue and collagen repair. Several studies have found low B6 levels in osteoporosis patients relative to same-age controls. Since this vitamin is inexpensive and remarkably safe at effective levels (50 mg once or twice a day), it is wise to supplement it along with magnesium.

10. Exercise

Bone building responds to exercise. Immobilising an arm in a sling for a prolonged period will result in bone mass loss in that arm. Immobilization in bed will result in bone loss throughout the skeleton. Astronauts, in a so-called gravity-free (actually, gravity balanced by centrifugal force) environment will begin losing calcium within a couple of days. Mineralized

---

Typical osteoporosis treatment programme

Diet Leafy green and other vegetables emphasized. Avoid all 'sodas' and limit red meat to 3 or fewer times per week. Limit alcohol use.

Vitamin D 350-400 i.u. daily

Vitamin C 2,000 mg/day in divided doses

Betacarotene 15 mg/day (equiv. to 25,000 i.u. of vitamin A)

Zinc 15-30 mg/day

Calcium 800-1000 mg/day by diet and/or supplements

Magnesium 300 mg/day

Oestrogen Use in minimum doses 3 weeks/month as needed for vaginal dryness. Do not use if contraindicated for any reason. Often not needed for osteoporosis treatment.

Progesterone Natural progesterone cream (e.g. Pro-Gest or equivalent creams) applied daily during the last two weeks of oestrogen use or 3 weeks/month if oestrogen not used. Use one-half of a 2-oz jar per month for 3 months. Later, one-third of a jar per month may suffice, as determined by serial BMD tests.

Exercise 12-20 minutes daily, or ½ hour 3 times/week.

No cigarettes.

Report any occurrence of vaginal bleeding.

---

bone (hydroxyapatite) is a crystalline structure and, as such, will respond to physical stress just as other crystalline structures do. In particular, any force tending to distort the crystalline arrangement generates an electric voltage, called the piezoelectric effect, producing a small electric current (discovered by Pierre Curie in 1883). This also happens in mineralized bone and may explain the wondrous ability of osteoclast and osteoblast action in constructing and reinforcing bone trabeculae along lines best suited for maximum strength and physical efficiency. When viewed microscopically, trabeculae remind one of the vaulted chambers and flying buttresses of the best Gothic churches.

Our modern day, labour saving devices and engine powered travel have greatly reduced the exercise previously experienced in everyday living. This lack of exercise diminishes the stimuli that promote bone strength. This, along with nutritional deficiencies, is probably the primary reason for the decrease in bone mineralization now evident. When bone mineral density is compared between present-day skeletons and those buried two centuries ago, as reported recently in *The Lancet*, the 'ancient' bones showed better BMD results than 'modern' bones.[26]

The form of exercise beneficial to bone is relatively unimportant as long as it imposes some exercise against resistance. Bone building simply does not occur in the absence of physical stress on bones. In advanced osteoporosis, however, some care must be given to avoid excessive force that could increase the risk of fracture.

Factors deleterious to bone

Just as attention must be paid to factors that promote good bones, so must one pay attention to factors that are deleterious to bone. Following is such a list.

1. The protein problem

Protein is essential for tissue growth and repair, and for enzyme synthesis, nucleic acids, neurotransmitters, and some hormones (e.g. insulin). For many years, science endorsed the concept of eating large amounts (120-185 gm/day) of protein, based on the theory of Liebig (early nineteenth century) that muscle protein was actually consumed by activity and must be replaced constantly. The fact that large intake of protein is unnecessary was first suggested by Chittenden in 1905. However, it is only recently that science agrees that protein requirements for adults are generally about 40-60 grams (or 1.5-2 oz) per day.[27]

If one eats more protein than required for nutritional purposes, it is not stored by the body (as fat is, for example) but must be excreted. Excess protein is catabolized and waste products are excreted in the urine. The renal excretion of protein waste products increases the urinary excretion of calcium. The ratio between calcium ingested and calcium lost in urine is called the *calcium balance*. A high intake of protein creates a negative calcium balance (i.e., more is lost than was ingested). Homeostatic requirements of a stable serum calcium level result in calcium being mobilized from bone to replace the calcium lost. This is the prime reason why vegetarians generally have better bones than those whose diets include meat in the style of the standard US diet.

In calculating protein intake, it is important to consider the protein content of various dietary components. The following list may be helpful.

Most meats . . . . approximately 25% protein
Chicken, turkey, cheese and fish . . . . 25-30% protein

Beans, peas and nuts. . . . . approximately 10-12% protein
Other vegetables . . . . range from 3.5-10% protein
One egg (egg white). . . . . 0.22 oz of protein; same as one bagel

2. Diuretics

Diuretics increase urine volume and are used extensively in medicine to treat oedema, congestive heart disease, or water retention from any cause. The use of diuretics correlates with increased fracture risk. A number of diuretics cause increased urinary excretion of minerals. Furosemide (Lasix) is the most common diuretic prescribed; it is also the one that promotes the greatest loss of calcium, thus a potential cause of osteoporosis. Other diuretics (e.g. thiazides) retain calcium but tend also to increase one's fracture risk by causing nocturnal urination which, among the elderly, increases the risk of accidental falls in the bathroom.

A better approach to water retention problems is by diet, if possible. If diuretics must be used, it is wise to choose those that do not increase calcium loss.

3. Antibiotics

Broad-spectrum antibiotics kill friendly intestinal bacteria that make vitamin K for us. Vitamin K is a bone-building factor. Long term or frequent courses of antibiotics result in low vitamin K levels and thereby interfere with bone building. If antibiotics must be used in such a manner, it is wise to supplement vitamin K and replenish friendly colon bacteria such as L. acidolphilus.

4. Fluoride

For some years, fluoride enthusiasts claimed fluoride is good for bones. The fact is that fluoride may slightly increase the X-ray appearance of bone mass but the resultant bone is of inferior quality and actually increases the risk of hip fracture. This is found not only in fluoride doses used in osteoporosis 'therapy' (i.e. 15-20 mg/day),[28-30] but also in doses obtained in fluoridated communities (i.e., 3-5 mg/day).[31-34] Fluoride is a potent enzyme inhibitor and, in bone, causes pathologic changes leading to increased risk of fracture. Fluoride, in all forms including toothpastes, should be avoided.

5. Metabolic acidosis

Metabolic acidosis refers to metabolic processes that would tend to increase the acidity (lower pH) of blood. It is necessary for the body to maintain blood pH within very narrow limits. Corrective homeostatic mechanisms include the use of calcium as a buffer. Cigarette smokers, for example, develop emphysema, or chronic obstructive pulmonary disease, leading to retained lung carbon dioxide and to increased serum carbonic acid. The body's response to the acidosis threat is to buffer the excess acid with calcium, usually taken from bone for the purpose.

6. Alcohol abuse

Whether from specific alcohol toxicity to bone, magnesium loss, or other nutritional deficiency, osteoporosis is rampant among alcoholics. A history of more-than-modest alcohol use is a potent risk factor for osteoporosis.

7. Hyperthyroidism

Hyperthyroidism, especially that resulting from excessive L-thyroxin supplementation, accelerates bone resorption and thus promotes osteoporosis, presumably by stimulating osteoclast activity. Persons receiving L-thyroxin supplements should routinely be checked with TSH tests to prevent this risk of bone loss.

Conclusion

Having summarized the various factors required for healthy, strong bones and the factors deleterious to bones, it is important that the central thesis of this chapter be restated:

> **Postmenopausal osteoporosis is a disease of inadequate osteoblast-mediated new bone formation secondary to progesterone deficiency. Progesterone restores osteoblast function. Natural progesterone hormone is an essential factor in the prevention and proper treatment of osteoporosis.**

In men, it should be added, testosterone fulfills the same function as progesterone. When all the right factors are present, bone building continues throughout life.

A programme for preventing or treating osteoporosis utilizing diet, a few nutritional supplements, exercise, and progesterone is described on p83 above: for more details on progesterone dosage, see pp117-119.

12

Progesterone and cancer

B REAST CANCER AND ENDOMETRIAL CANCER are two cancers that are related in some way or other to sex hormones. They occur in tissues sensitive to these hormones. Unopposed oestrogen is the only known cause of endometrial cancer though there may well be other factors involved. Oestrogen, or at least one or more of the various oestrogens, are thought to contribute to breast cancer incidence.[1-5] It is therefore appropriate to review the role of the other gonadal hormone, progesterone.

In general, cancer is the abnormal growth of cells in our bodies sufficient to kill us if left untreated. All cancer originates as a change of a normal cell. The cell *increases* its rate of multiplication and *loses* the quality of differentiation. Normally, most cells replicate themselves continually at a rate synchronous with normal growth and repair. Each cell (with the exception of ova and sperm) contains a full complement of chromosomes; yet each develops in a manner specific for its purpose in the body. When it becomes a cancer cell, it multiplies faster than it should and loses normal differentiation. In that sense it becomes a more primitive cell, growing at its own rate in a manner more avaricious than the normal cells from whence it came.

The actual mechanism by which cancer is caused is still speculative. There are two competing but not mutually exclusive theories. One, the *genetic* theory, proposes that cancer is the product of chromosomal DNA damage induced by radiation, viruses, or toxins. The body combats this by chromosomal repair mechanisms, but, as one's life progresses, the accumulated bits of damage to various genomes increase over time. Thus, the incidence of cancer increases with age. It is thought that, for a cell to become cancerous, five or more genomes must be damaged. Factors that interfere or impede repair mechanisms will predispose one to cancer.

A more recent *epigenetic* theory holds that certain toxic environments within the cell cytoplasm can stimulate a latent ability of otherwise undamaged chromosomes to switch to a more primitive mode of survival in response to the epigenetic threat. This latter theory suggests that (1) maintaining a healthy intra-cellular environment will prevent cancer, and that (2) correcting a toxic intra-cellular environment may lead to successful non-toxic treatment for cancer. Evidence against the genetic theory and/or favouring the epigenetic theory includes the following:

- Under the same risk exposure, only some people develop cancer
- Under similar exposure to known carcinogens, different individuals develop cancer at different tissue sites.
- In humans and other animals (e.g., hamsters) exposed to known carcinogens, cancer can be prevented by agents such as betacarotene, or vitamin C, etc.
- In cell culture tests, cancer induced by known carcinogens can be reversed and eliminated by improving the nutrient quality of the cell culture.
- In humans with advanced cancer, survival time is often increased by high-dose vitamin C.
- Similarly, changes in patient attitude seem to extend survival time.
- In humans, 'spontaneous' remissions and apparent cures may result simply from dietary changes.

Further, there is the thought that some factors operate as *initiators* and others as *promoters* of cancer. An initiatior might be one that creates the damage to the genome or is a toxin within the cytoplasm; and a promoter may be one that impedes repair mechanisms. Or, an initiator may be a factor that will eventually cause cancer and a promoter is one that shortens the time interval between exposure to the carcinogen and the development of cancer. In the ultimate balance of conditions that keep cells healthy, the difference between initiator factors and promoter factors is quite subtle, it would seem.

Progesterone, oestrogen and breast cancer

Both breast cancer and endometrial cancer are health risks that tend to surface in women at a time in their lives when oestrogen dominance is likely. In the case of breast cancer, consider the following observations:

- Breast cancer is more likely to occur in premenopausal women with normal or high oestrogen levels and low progesterone levels.[6] This situation may occur in early adult life in a few women but is quite common after age 35 or so when anovulatory periods tend to occur. It also occurs after menopause when women are given oestrogen supplements without progesterone.
- Among premenopausal women, breast cancer recurrence or late metas-

tases after mastectomy for breast cancer is more common when surgery has been performed during the first half of the menstrual cycle (when oestrogen is the dominant hormone) than when surgery has been performed during the latter half of their menstrual cycle (when progesterone is dominant).[7]

- Tamoxifen (a weak oestrogenic compound that competes with natural oestrogen at receptor sites) is commonly prescribed to women after breast cancer surgery for the purpose of preventing recurrence of their cancer.
- Pregnancy occurring before age 25-30 is known to have a protective effect.
- Only the first, full-term, early pregnancy conveys protection. Women having their first pregnancies before age 18 have approximately one-third the risk of women bearing the first child after age 35. Interrupted pregnancies (induced or spontaneous abortions) do not afford protection and may, in fact, increase the risk of breast cancer.
- Women without children are at a higher risk than those with one or more children.
- In women subjected to oophorectomy (removal of both ovaries) prior to age 40, their risk of breast cancer is significantly reduced.
- Protective effects of early oophorectomy is negated by administration of oestrogen.
- Treatment of males with oestrogen (for prostatic cancer or after transsexual surgery) is associated with an increased risk of breast cancer.
- Recently, industrial pollutants having potent oestrogenic effects, called xenooestrogens, are being recognized as a pervasive environmental threat, likely to be a contributing factor in the incidence of breast cancer.[8]

Such correlations strongly suggest that oestrogen, especially if unopposed by progesterone, is somehow related to the development of breast cancer. The cancer protective benefit of progesterone is clearly indicated by the prospective study in which premenopausal women with low progesterone levels were found to have 5.4 times the risk of developing premenopausal breast cancer and a 10-fold increase in deaths from all malignant neoplasms compared to those with normal progesterone levels.[6]

It should be recalled that not all oestrogens are equivalent in their actions on breast tissue. Among the three major natural oestrogens, oestradiol is the most stimulating to breast tissue, oestrone is second, and oestriol by far the least. During pregnancy, oestriol is the dominant oestrogen, being produced in great quantities by the placenta while ovarian production of oestradiol and oestrone is quiescent. Since all oestrogens compete for the same receptor sites, it is probable that sufficient oestriol impedes the carcinogenic effects of oestradiol and/or oestrone. In a remarkable paper by Lemon et al in the *JAMA* of 27 June 1966,[9] it was reported that women with breast cancer excreted 30-60% *less* oestriol than non-cancer controls; and that remission of cancer in patients receiving endocrine therapy occurred only in those whose oestriol quotient *rose*. That is, low levels of oestriol relative to oestradiol and oestrone correlate with increased risk of breast cancer and higher levels of oestriol from endocrine treatment correlate with remission of cancer. Further, rodent studies show that oestrone and oestradiol are carcinogenic for breast cancer in male or castrated females whereas oestriol is not.

Prevention and treatment of breast cancer

Much confusion reigns over the relationship of sex hormones to breast cancer. Most experienced clinicians understand very well that oestrogen is a promoter of breast cancer, and they also understand that progesterone balances or opposes undesirable side effects of oestrogen. For reasons which are not clear, in treating breast cancer conventional medicine has ignored the cancer-protective effects of natural progesterone, despite the many studies that offer evidence (see 'Using progesterone cream' below). Even though progesterone (or more likely a progestin) has been used in hormone replacement therapy (HRT) to offset or oppose oestrogen's role in promoting endometrial cancer, progesterone has not been widely recognised for its similar role in preventing breast cancer.

Testing the effect of progesterone

One good way to test progesterone's effect on breast cancer incidence would be to measure oestrogen and progesterone levels in a large number of women and follow their lives to observe any correlation in the subsequent incidence of breast cancer. This has been done. In 1981, Johns Hopkins researchers published their results showing that the breast cancer incidence was *5.4 times greater* in women with *low* progesterone than in women who had good progesterone levels. This difference remained true despite differences in a woman's age of menarche, age of menopause, history of oral contraceptive use, history of benign breast disease, or her age at the birth of her first child.[10]

Further, when the incidence of all types of neoplasms was looked at, they found that the incidence was 10-fold higher in women with low progesterone levels compared to women with good progesterone levels.

A second test would be to measure progesterone levels in women at the time when they are diagnosed as having breast cancer. This too has been done. Dr David Zava tested oestrogen and progesterone levels in breast tissue specimens from several thousand women who had undergone breast cancer surgery.[11] Almost universally they revealed oestrogen dominance — i.e. a relative deficiency in progesterone. The one exception was a woman whose tissue revealed a total lack of progesterone receptors, a rare genetic defect. As might be expected, the course of her disease was brief and fatal.

Another relevant factor would be the survival rate after breast cancer surgery of women with differing progesterone levels. At least 10 retrospective studies have been carried out which show a longer disease-free period or overall survival advantage to resection of a cycling woman's breast cancer when done in the early luteal phase (when progesterone is presumed to be at its highest), compared to surgery performed during the proliferative phase (when progesterone is very low). William J.M. Hrushesky reviewed these data in 1996 and listed 7 known mechanisms of action whereby progesterone inhibits breast cancer cell growth and/or metastases.[12]

In a 20-year prospective study published in 1996 in the *British Journal of Cancer*, Dr P. E. Mohr et al reported that women with a progesterone level of 4 ng/ml or more at the time of their breast cancer surgery had a significantly better survival rate at 18 years than those with a lower serum level of progesterone. This was especially clear in nodepositive women. Among women with good progesterone levels at the time of surgery, approximately 65% were surviving 18 years later, when among women with low progesterone levels at the time of surgery, only about 35% were surviving.[13]

Cell death is life-giving

The multiple mechanisms by which progesterone protects against breast cancer, and oestrogen increases the risk of breast cancer, have been reviewed in an illuminating paper by chronobiologist Dr William Hrushesky.[12] In addition to the increased cell proliferation caused by oestrogen, Dr Hrushesky describes a number of other important mechanisms. Of particular interest is apoptosis (pronounced a-po-toe-sis) or programmed cell suicide. With the exception of nerve and muscle cells, all the cells of the body are constantly being replaced with newly made cells. This requires that normal cells live only for a specified period of time, and then die as new cells come along to replace them.

This death of old cells is necessary for continued good health. Old skin cells are shed, as are the lining cells of respiratory organs and the gastrointestinal system. In the breast, however, the old cells that undergo apoptosis are consumed by macrophages (special white blood cells). *It is now well understood by cancer specialists that if the apoptosis of these older cells is delayed, it increases their risk of becoming cancer cells.*

There are a number of ways in which oestrogen influences apoptosis and other cellular actions toward cancer, and several ways in which progesterone has the opposite, anti-cancer effect.

1   Oestradiol, one of the forms of oestrogen, increases cell proliferation and promotes delayed or inhibited apoptosis. Both of these characteristics promote cancer. Progesterone *decreases* both characteristics.

2   Unopposed oestrogen compromises cellular activities in the immune system, specifically natural killer cell activity and the working of interleukin-2, both of which help destroy early cancer cells. An adequate level of progesterone *promotes* these actions.

3   The metastasis (spread) of cancer cells depends partly on the permeability of blood vessels (their ability to allow substances to pass through their walls). Progesterone *reduces* blood vessel permeability, and thus helps protect against cancer cell metastasis.

Dr Hrushesky's work has also shed important light on the issue of timing in breast cancer surgery, making it clear that women who have surgery at a time in their menstrual cycle when progesterone levels are high have a lower recurrence rate than women who have surgery when oestrogen levels are high and/or progesterone levels are low.

Beyond these influences, there is now even more fundamental research which links oestrogen dominance to breast cancer at the genetic level.

Getting down to the gene level

If their genes are damaged — for example by radiation, toxins or virus attack — normal cells can develop into cancer cells. Certain mutated genes called oncogenes produce products that allow excessive cell proliferation or delayed apoptosis, and can transform the cell into a cancer cell. Other genes, known to be tumour suppressor genes, inhibit cell division or stimulate apoptosis, and prevent cancer. *One's risk of cancer depends in large part on the activity of oncogenes versus tumour suppressor genes.*

Researchers have grown cultures of cancer cells and then treated them with oestrogen and progesterone.[14] They found that when they added oestradiol to the culture in concentrations consistent with human levels, oncogenes were activated and cancer growth was promoted. When they added progesterone in concentrations consistent with normal physiologic levels, they found that tumour suppressor genes were stimulated and oncogenes were suppressed, which stopped cancer growth. This illustrates at least one gene-related mechanism that connects oestradiol to cancer promotion.

Corroboration of these findings comes from Dr Ercole Cavalieri, who has been working for thirty years on finding the connection between genes and breast cancer.[15] Through meticulous and extremely complex biochemical sleuthing, Dr Cavalieri has tracked the metabolism of oestrogens through several pathways.

He found that most pathways lead to harmless products that are excreted by the body. However, one pathway leads to an oestrogen by-product that causes carcinogenic mutation in genes. I believe this constitutes a smoking gun regarding oestrogen's role in promoting cancer at the genetic level.

It is important to note that of the three major types of human oestrogen — oestrone, oestradiol and oestriol — only oestrone and oestradiol follow the metabolic pathway that creates this cancer-causing substance. Oestriol does not participate in these metabolic pathways. It cannot become a catechol oestrogen, so it is simply not carcinogenic. Nor are the phytooestrogens, the plant-based oestrogens from soy, wild yams and other sources. The risk comes only from oestrone and oestradiol.

Other carcinogens are known to stimulate, accelerate or intensify the production of these harmful oestrogen products, especially during one's embryo life. These include pesticides and solvents, the manufacturing by-product dioxin, and the synthetic oestrogen DES.

It is appalling to contrast these scientific findings with the conventional practice of prescribing oestrogen replacement therapy (ORT) alone to women without a uterus, or hormone replacement therapy (HRT) using oestrogen with progestins. Progestins are *not* the same as progesterone, and they do *not* provide the vital intracellular message that stimulates tumour-suppressor genes that fight cancer and suppresses the oncogenes that regulate it.

Natural defences against genetic mutation

Mother Nature has created a series of defences against carcinogenic mutations in genes.

For example, the change to harmful oestrogen by-products can be partially prevented if your diet contains enough of the proper fatty acids and avoids harmful oils such as the transfatty hydrogenated oils. Sulphur-containing amino acids such as cysteine and methionine also block the harmful path: they are found in almost all fresh, whole foods, but are especially high in garlic, onions, cruciferous vegetables such as broccoli and cauliflower, and beans.

Using progesterone cream

We know that there are three characteristics by which cancer cells differ from normal cells. These are (1) rate of proliferation, (2) degree of differentiation, and (3) rate of apoptosis (programmed cell suicide). In brief, cancer cells multiply more rapidly and are less differentiated than normal cells, and they do not die on time. Keeping tissues healthy (tissue homeostasis) results from cells having an appropriate proliferation rate, full differentiation, and dying on time.

It should not be surprising that sex hormones have a role in all three of these processes in breast cells. Breasts in females obviously change at puberty when oestrogen and progesterone production rises. The action of oestradiol (E2) and progesterone on cell multiplication (proliferation) in breast cells was beautifully demonstrated in an important 1995 study by Chang, de Lignieres et al. which tested the effects of transdermal (via the skin) hormone applications on human breast milk duct epithelial cells — from which cancer is known to arise — in healthy young women planning to undergo minor breast surgery for benign breast disease.[16] In this study, the women were divided into four groups. For 8-10 days before surgery,

Group A applied oestradiol cream (1.5mg) daily;

Group B applied progesterone cream (25mg) daily;

Group C applied a combination of oestradiol and progesterone (half doses of each) daily; and

Group D applied a placebo cream.

At surgery, biopsies were obtained for measuring oestradiol and progesterone concentrations, and for tests of cell proliferation rates. Blood plasma hormone levels were also measured.

The results indicated that in comparison with the placebo cream, oestradiol cream increased oestradiol concentration in breast cells by over 100% and the progesterone cream increased progesterone concentration in breast cells by 100%. The combination cream resulted in a 50% increase of both hormones. This clearly demonstrates that both hormones are well absorbed transdermally, and accumulate in target tissues in the same manner as endogenous hormones.

Just as clear was the effect of these hormones on cell proliferation rates.

Dr Lee's Basic Breast Cancer Prevention Programme

1   **Limit consumption of** sugar, refined carbohydrates (pasta, white bread, white rice), trans-fatty acids (hydrogenated oils, margarines, fried foods), and oestrogen-rich foods such as feed lot meat and cows' milk. **Increase your consumption of** foods with sulphated amino acids, such as beans, onions, and garlic.

2   To prevent higher risk of cancer in our children, women (and men) contemplating pregnancy should **avoid xenobiotics found in food containing pesticides and insecticide residue, and learn to eat organically grown food. Avoid processed foods** as much as possible because they contain harmful dyes and a potpourri of other chemicals with unknown effects. **Also avoid all types of pesticides, herbicides and fungicides, including household sprays and lawn and garden chemicals**. This is also an important step for prevention of breast cancer and prostate cancer in adults.

3   Women must become aware that **hormone imbalance starts progressively earlier in industrialized countries**. Progesterone levels may become deficient by age 25 or 30, and this deficiency affects about 50% of women by age 35 in the US, thus creating oestrogen dominance. When hormone level testing or symptoms indicate oestrogen dominance, progesterone should be supplemented.

4   **Foreign progesterone-like prescription compounds such as those found in Provera and in birth con trol pills should be avoided** and not confused with real progesterone. Birth control pills play an important role in creating early hormone imbalances, and should be avoided if at all possible. There is no reason to believe that progestins such as Provera are as beneficial as real progesterone when it comes to preventing cancer.

5   Even after menopause, oestrogen (oestrone) is still being created by cella in body fat. **Oestrogen supplementation should only be used if indicated by vaginal dryness or thinning, night sweats, or hot flashes**. The correct dose is the least dose that prevents these symptoms. Oestriol is safer in regard to breast cancer than oestrone or oestradiol.

6   **Prescriptions for unopposed oestrogen should be banned**. No woman should ever be given oestrogen without progesterone, even if she doesn't have a uterus or ovaries. When oestrogen supplementation is indicated, it should be preceded by progesterone supplementation, and the oestrogen dose should be kept as low as possible.

Oestradiol increased the cell proliferation rate by 230% whereas progesterone decreased it by more than 400%. The oestradiol/progesterone combination cream maintained the normal proliferation rate. Again, this is clear evidence that that unoppoed oestradiol stimulated hyperproliferation of breast epithelial cells, and progesterone protects against this. And since oestradiol and oestrone can be converted one to the other in the liver and intestines, it is fair to include unopposed oestrone as a potential danger too.

The blood plasma tests, on the other hand, showed no measurable increase of progesterone concentration. This is an excellent illustration of the fact that bioavailable progesterone is carried in blood but not in blood plasma. This simple fact nullifies all previous claims, based on plasma or serum testing, that progesterone is not well absorbed through the skin.

This double blind, randomised, placebo controlled *in vivo* study proves that both oestradiol and progesterone are well absorbed transdermally. Furthermore it shows that oestradiol stimulates proliferation of breast epithelial cells, whereas progesterone reduces it. Since excessive cell proliferation (hyperplasia) is a recognised hallmark of potential cancer development, this study strongly suggests that oestradiol increases that risk, while progesterone protects against it.

It is also important for illustrating that plasma levels do not adequately reflect transdermal progesterone absorption. We now know that saliva hormone assay is far superior to 'blood tests' in this matter.

The evidence is strong that unopposed oestradiol and oestrone are carcinogenic for breasts, and both progesterone and oestriol, the two major hormones throughout pregnancy, are protective against breast cancer. One is left to wonder why supplementation with these two beneficial and safe hormones is not used routinely for women whenever hormone supplementation seems indicated. There should be no difficulty in measuring progesterone levels and urinary oestriol levels to determine who might be at increased risk of breast cancer and who would benefit from supplementation. Both hormones are available and are relatively inexpensive. Why have they been neglected by contemporary medical practice in favour of synthetic substitutes? A probable answer derives from the medical-industrial complex now dominating medical practice and will be presented in Chapter 16.

Progesterone and endometrial cancer

It is generally acknowledged that the only known cause of endometrial cancer is unopposed oestrogen. Here, again, oestradiol and oestrone are the culprits. When given to postmenopausal women, oestrogen supplements for five years increase the risk of endometrial cancer 6-fold, and longer term use increases it to 15-fold. In premenopausal women, endometrial cancer is extremely rare except during the 5-10 years before menopause when oestrogen dominance is common.

The addition of natural progesterone during these years would significantly reduce the incidence of endometrial cancer (as well as breast cancer, as noted above).

Endometrial cancer is a relatively safe cancer in that it generally shows itself early by abnormal vaginal bleeding and it metastasizes relatively late in its course. It is cured by hysterectomy performed prior to metastases. Women treated by hysterectomy for endometrial cancer are advised, however, to avoid 'hormones' forever. Like patients with history of breast cancer, they face a future of progressive osteoporosis, vaginal atrophy and recurrent urinary tract infections without recourse to hormonal therapy. These are the women for whom I first began using natural progesterone therapy. Not only did progesterone reverse their osteoporosis and, in many, it corrected their vaginal atrophy, but none, to my knowledge, have ever developed cancer of any sort. (If vaginal atrophy remains a problem, intravaginal oestriol would be the treatment of choice. See Chapter 9.) Further, among those with intact uteri, none have ever developed any uterine problems of any kind. The evidence is overwhelming that natural progesterone is safe and only oestradiol, oestrone, and the various synthetic oestrogens and progestins are to be avoided to reduce one's risk of endometrial cancer.

Ovarian cancer

Your ovaries protect your health: hang on to them if you can. They're unpredictable, they're complicated, and they're good for your health and longevity.

A woman's ovaries are the anatomical equivalent of a man's testicles. A man's testicles are a source of hormone-generated energy and libido, and a woman's ovaries serve a similar function. And just as removing a man's testicles is castration, removing a woman's ovaries is known as female castration. I'm not making this up. That is the medical term for removing a woman's ovaries and it carries all the physical results and implications that go with that loaded word.

The effect of castration upon a woman is just as profound as it is on a man, although some doctors may be adamant that it will solve all of a woman's problems. It's possible that those doctors are correct in their assertion, in the same sense that castrating a man will solve all of his 'problems.'

Hysterectomy, in which the uterus is removed but the ovaries are left intact, will ultimately result in functional castration. Removing the uterus will severely restrict blood flow to the ovaries, and within a few years the ovaries will no longer function. Many women believe that this complete loss of ovarian function will occur anyway as a result of menopause, but this is not true. Normally, the ovaries are functional well after menopause, producing the hormone androstenedione, which can be converted to oestrogen in fat cells.

A woman who is castrated and no longer makes any appreciable amounts of oestrogen, progesterone and androstenedione will often become depressed, have little to no libido, and with the addition of some Premarin (a synthetic oestrogen) prescribed by her doctor, she will retain water and probably will be a little anxious as well. She will also increase her risk of osteoporosis and heart disease even if she is put on replacement hormones. If she is put just on Premarin and Provera (PremPro or PremPhase), the standard medical practice, her risk of breast cancer will rise, especially after five years. Even if she supplements with all of the steroid hormones, they will not be as well regulated as they would have been by her ovaries.

The vast majority of female castrations, also called oophorectomies, are unnecessary. One reason that doctors tend to be eager to remove the ovaries is that they fear ovarian cancer, and see oophorectomy as preventive medicine. Even though ovarian cancer is relatively rare, it is very frightening to those who have been through it, because it is difficult to diagnose until it is fairly advanced, and has a very low rate of remission in response to conventional medicine.

Ovarian cancer isn't easy to diagnose early

Ovarian cancer accounts for nearly 20% of gynaecologic cancers, and ranks fifth in cancer fatalities in women. In the US it causes about 13,500 deaths per year, or 5.3% of the 254,000 annual deaths from cancer among women. Most ovarian cancer occurs in menopausal women who are around the age of 50.

The best method your physician has of diagnosing ovarian cancer is palpation (feeling it with the hands) during a pelvic exam. Younger women will frequently have enlarged or 'functional' cysts on their ovaries, and most doctors will give the cysts six weeks to disappear — which they usually do — before doing exploratory surgery.

Menopausal women in their fifties have smaller ovaries that normally aren't detectable with palpation, so the presence of a larger ovary in a menopausal woman can be cause for concern.

Benign (non-cancerous) ovarian cysts are very common in premenopausal women, and as the cysts go through the process of 'resolving' or dissolving, they can create all manner of symptoms, which greatly complicates the diagnosis of ovarian cancer. Jesse Hanley, M.D., reports that the symptoms of ovarian cancer can include abdominal pain and bloating, sharp pains and cramps, a feeling of indigestion and, sometimes, irregular bleeding. But she notes that between erratic ovaries that ovulate some months and not others (a common occurrence in premenopausal women) and an occasionally fussy uterus that cramps, most women become accustomed to sporadic aches and pains in that part of the body. As a result, the symptoms of ovarian cancer may go unnoticed until it has affected other parts of the pelvic cavity.

Symptoms associated with excessive or deficient oestrogen, progesterone, or antrogens (male hormones), can also be symptoms of ovarian cancer, because the tumour may create an excess or deficiency of these hormones. Yet these are symptoms that could easily be dismissed by a premenopausal woman whose hormones are fluctuating. In most cases, these types of symptoms are not cause for alarm until you are well into your menopausal years, in which case you should see your doctor about them.

If you have a family history of ovarian cancer or other reproductive cancers, or if you have some of the risk factors mentioned below, it's probably worth getting a yearly AMAS (anti-malignan antibody in serum) test starting at around age 40, to rule out a malignancy.

The rarity of ovarian cancer makes it difficult to accumulate enough cases to research its cause or causes. It is however generally considered a hormone-dependent cancer, along with breast, endometrial, and prostate cancer.

What we know about the causes of ovarian cancer

Oestrogen is a likely suspect, and so are birth control pills and fertility drugs.

In 1995, an important report described the correlation between oestrogen replacement therapy and fatal ovarian cancer. In this study, 240,073 peri- and postmenopausal women, who first enrolled in the study in 1982, were followed for at least 7 years during which time 436 of them died of ovarian cancer. It was found that the incidence of ovarian cancer increased with the duration of oestrogen replacement therapy. Among those who used ERT for 6 years or more, the risk of fatal ovarian cancer increased by 72%, relative to those who had never used it. This increased risk was not modified by any other potential factors.[17]

It should be noted that this report concerns women receiving unopposed oestrogen (ERT), and provides no data on those who receive hormone replacement therapy (HRT), which also includes progestins or progesterone.

The relationship between hormones and ovarian cancer has also been studied by molecular biologists who test the effect of hormones on cancer cell cultures. In a major (but as yet unpublished) study, researchers B. Formby and T. S. Wiley of the Sansum Medical Research Foundation in Santa Barbara, CA, have done just that with cultures of breast, ovarian, endometrial, and prostate cancer cells. The results are stunningly clear. In all these tissues, the addition of oestradiol (a natural oestrogen) greatly increased the growth of the cancer cells, whereas the addition of progesterone stopped their growth.

Fertility drugs can cause ovarian cancer

One of the causes of the increasing rate of ovarian cancer is the widespread use of fertility drugs that stimulate the ovaries to mature follicles. The longer the drugs are used, the more the risk of ovarian cancer increases. One study found that using fertility drugs increased ovarian cancer risk three times, but in women who never gave birth and were treated with fertility drugs the risk was increased 27-fold.[18] Other studies have shown that women who are infertile, and women who delay childbearing, also have a higher risk of ovarian cancer, so a woman who uses fertility drugs may be significantly increasing an already elevated risk.

Dr. Hanley is particularly concerned that the increasing use of fertility drugs by thousands of women, combined with oestrogen dominance, may create an epidemic of ovarian cancer in the next few decades.

Other causes of ovarian cancer

Some researchers believe that the ovulation process causes cellular trauma that stimulates cells in the ovary to divide, leading to malignancy. This hypothesis is supported by the statistics which show that the more full-term pregnancies a woman has had, the lower her risk of ovarian cancer.

Pregnancy is a time when the ovaries get a rest for nine months. As a result, a woman who has had several full-term pregnancies has ovulated less frequently in her lifetime than a woman who hasn't had children, while a woman who has not had a full-term pregnancy ovulates continuously, every month. In addition, during pregnancy progesterone levels are very high, and progesterone is protective against reproductive cancers.

Statistically, we know that your risk of ovarian cancer increases if you have used birth control pills; if you have a relative who has had it; if your consumption of dairy protucts is high; and if you use talcum powder. (It is thought that the powder, which contains toxins such as heavy metals, actually migrates up the vagina, through the cervix, into the uterus and onto the ovaries.)

Given everything we've discussed, it seems clear and reasonable to me that ovarian cancer which is not directly caused by fertility drugs or birth control pills, is most likely to be primarily related to unopposed oestrogen and a deficiency in progesterone. I believe that the proper medical care of women should include a sensitivity to the problem of oestrogen dominance and progesterone deficiency, which has become epidemic during early adult life. Ovarian cancer is just one of the diseases that we may be able to prevent through appropriate supplementation with natural progesterone in women with oestrogen dominance.

Conclusion

Breast and endometrial cancer are two of the greatest fears, along with osteoporosis, that women face as they approach menopause. These fears, under present circumstances, are well warranted. However, they need not be. When the cause of any given cancer is known, prevention becomes a reality. Lung cancer, for example, can be almost completely prevented by never smoking cigarettes. Among many cancers, the cause is still unknown. However, for breast and endometrial cancer, a great deal is known about its major hormonal factors. The only mystery is, why hasn't this information permeated the halls of contemporary medicine? The carcinogenic effects of unopposed oestradiol and oestrone, and the anti-cancer benefits of oestriol and progesterone are well established for these two cancers.

Because of its many benefits, its great safety, and particularly its ability to oppose the carcinogenic effects of oestrogens, natural progesterone deserves far more attention and application than generally given in the prevention and care of women's health problems today.

13

Women's heart disease and hormones

Y OU CAN CAUSE OR HELP PREVENT cardiovascular disease, depending on the hormone you choose. I'm about to give you a lot of seemingly discouraging statistics about women and heart disease, but stay with me: by the end of this chapter you'll know a lot about how to prevent heart disease.

The rate of death from heart disease in the US has gradually declined over the past 20 years, but that decline has been much steeper for men than for women, and from 1992-1995 death rates from heart attacks in women increased. Until a few years ago, doctors didn't take heart disease symptoms in women very seriously: one out of three of them didn't even know it is the leading cause of death in women, more than all other causes of death combined. Eventually, with age, about 50% of women die of heart disease.

Women are more likely to die of a first heart attack, and two-thirds of them have no previous symptoms, compared to only half of men who have no previous symptoms. Some people guess that the women do have previous symptoms, but either don't go to the doctor for them, or the doctor doesn't take them seriously. It is also possible that the cause or mechanism of women's heart problems is different in some way from that of men.

One year after a heart attack, 44% of women have died, as compared to only 27% of men. Although women tend to live about seven years longer than men, they spend twice as many years disabled before they die.

We don't know whether taking aspirin prevents heart disease in women. We do know that hysterectomy, with or without the removal of the ovaries, leads to a much greater risk of heart disease, and that this risk is somewhat, but not entirely, lessened by taking oestrogen.

Challenging hormone dogma

The prevailing dogma about women and heart disease has been that it increases rapidly after menopause, and the assumption is that this is due to oestrogen deficiency. However, Harvard researcher Meir Stampfer, M.D., recently presented a controversial paper at a menopause symposium in Florence, showing that a woman's increasing risk of heart disease is correlated with age, but not with menopause. What makes this intriguing to me is that his information was based on pre-1985 data, and more recent data shows that there is a correlation with menopause. Some research shows that women's risk of heart disease eventually exceeds that of men. Has something created a correlation between death from heart disease in women and menopause since 1986?

Women's symptoms point to spasms

It is oxidised LDL cholesterol that clogs the arteries and leads to a heart attack. However, only 50% of coronary artery disease deaths are associated with clogged arteries, and the majority of those are men. Autopsies show that plaque obstructed arteries in women are considerably less clogged than those of men, most often only 20 to 30% blockage, which is not sufficient to cause their deaths. Men, by contrast, tend to have more than 90% occlusion when they have a heart attack.

Chest pain is the most common symptom of heart disease and heart attack in both men and women, but women having a heart attack are more likely to complain of upper abdominal pain, difficulty breathing, nausea and fatigue. Syndrome X is a cluster of heart disease symptoms that almost exclusively affects menopausalwomen. The symptoms of women with Syndrome X include exertional angina (chest pain in response to exercise) and a positive response to diagnostic exercise testing, and yet they have clear coronary arteries.

Prior to menopause (surgical or otherwise) women may have what are considered to be heart disease risk factors such as high cholesterol and blood pressure, yet they rarely die of a heart attack. So how do women die of heart attacks after menopause? Perhaps we can take our clue from research done by Dr. Kent Hermsmeyer, and others.[1]

Provera makes arteries more prone to spasm

Hermsmeyer and his colleagues set out to study the effect of hormones on coronary artery spasm. They removed the ovaries from 12 rhesus monkeys to simulate menopause. Then six of the monkeys were put on oestradiol (an oestrogen) and natural progesterone, and six were put on oestradiol and the synthetic progestin medroxyprogesterone acetate or MPA (Provera). Four weeks later the monkeys were injected with a combination of serotonin plus a platelet extract (thromboxane A2) known to stimulate coronary artery spasm. The monkeys that were on MPA and oestrogen suffered from an unrelenting spasm that would have caused death had they not been injected with a drug that reversed the spasm. The monkeys that had been treated with oestradiol and natural progesterone showed very little coronary artery spasm.

These findings are echoed by work done at Wake Forest University's Bowman School of Medicine in Winston-Salem, NC, led by J. Koudy Williams.[2] Their research with monkeys, heart disease and hormones has shown that medroxyprogesterone 'can obliterate the beneficial effect of oestrogen therapy on the progression of coronary artery atherosclerosis', which is clogging of the arteries.

At London's National Heart and Lung Institute, in a study led by Peter Collins, women on different combinations of hormone replacement therapy were put on a treadmill.[3] Once again, those who were using natural progesterone with oestrogen could exercise significantly longer than those who took medroxyprogesterone.

My hypothesis is that the increased risk of cardiovascular disease now associated with menopause may not be due to relatively minor cholesterol plaque or to hormone deficiency *per se*, but to increased risk of coronary vasospasm caused by synthetic progestins such as medroxyprogesterone acetate used in HRT. This does not ignore the effects of aging and the other factors listed below, it points the finger at a dangerous drug.

There's absolutely no excuse for any doctor to prescribe Provera for HRT when we have this kind of data. HRT should include small, physiologic doses of transdermal natural progesterone, which will protect against coronary vasospasm, combined with very small amounts of oestrogen, when needed.

When it comes to optimal cardiovascular health, some women may benefit from a small amount of oestrogen. But it is quite probable that for many women, postmenopausal production of oestrone in fat cells may be sufficient when supplemented with natural progesterone.

An anti-spasm mineral

A deficiency of the mineral magnesium can greatly increase the chance of a coronary vasospasm, and it is also implicated in mitral valve prolapse. Magnesium deficiency is common but generally unrecognised in the US, and yet cardiovascular survival correlates with magnesium concentrations, and higher cardiovascular disease mortality correlates with magnesium-depleting factors such as diuretic usage, diabetes, digoxin therapy, alcohol, age, congestive heart failure, diarrhoea, and dietary deficiency.

A daily supplement of 300 to 400 mg of magnesium is good preventive medicine. It should be taken with no more than twice the amount of calcium for optimal absorption.

Other factors in heart disease

Homocysteine Homocysteine is a waste product of methionine that is normally converted into a safer compound for excretion in urine. If it isn't converted, it accumulates and contributes to heart disease. The B vitamins B6, B12 and folic acid play key roles in the conversion of homocysteine, and deficiency can cause high homocysteine levels. A good daily multi-vitamin will contain 50 mg of vitamin B6; 400 mcg of folic acid; and 1,000 mcg of vitamin B12.

Antioxidants In the Nurse's Questionnaire Study and the Harvard Men's Study, those whose intake of vitamin E equalled at least 100 IU experienced 35-50% fewer heart attacks, and a more recent study from Great Britain showed as much as a 70% reduced risk. Vitamin E is especially effective because it is fat-soluble and thus more likely to supply oxidation protection to fatty compounds such as cholesterol. In considering the potential benefit of water-soluble vitamin and mineral antioxidants it is probably wise to include vitamin C and selenium, also. I recommend daily: 400 IU of vitamin E, 200 mcg of selenium, and at least 500 mg twice daily of vitamin C.

Oils Many studies show the benefits of eating fish, nuts and seeds which contain heart-healthy oils, and olive oil. Avoid hydrogenated and unsaturated oils.

Veggies People who eat more fresh fruits and vegetables, and more fibre, have less heart disease.

Alcohol People who drink a moderate amount of alcohol have less heart disease.

Sugar and milk Eat a minimum of sugar and refined carbohydrates, and stay away from milk after puberty.

Iron Excess iron can promote oxidation reactions that increase the risk of heart disease. Unless you are anaemic, find a multivitamin without iron.

Exercise Moderate, enjoyable exercise greatly reduces heart disease risks.

Weight While true obesity increases the risk of heart disease, the moderate weight gain most women experience around menopause is not harmful.

14

Prostate problems and hormones

Now I want to address a subject that affects the majority of men by the time they reach the age of eighty.

Some years back, a handful of men called or wrote to tell me of their experience with progesterone, usually the result of handling progesterone cream while helping a woman apply it. They reported that their symptoms of prostate enlargement or benign prostatic hypertrophy (BPH) such as urinary urgency and frequency decreased considerably, and their sexual performance increased. Needless to say, this gave me much to think about.

Testosterone is only part of the picture

Since then, several men with prostate cancer have told me that their PSA (Prostate Specific Antigen) level — an indication of prostate cancer — decreased when they started using a daily dab of progesterone cream, and that they have had no progression of their prostate lesions since using the cream. One man called to say his bone metastases are now no longer visible by Mayo Clinic X-ray tests.

Though I retired from active practice ten years ago, six of my former patients with early prostate cancer have been using progesterone cream (along with diet, some vitamin and mineral supplements, and saw palmetto) for about five years. All report their cancer has shown no progression.

The wrong treatment all these years

Since Huggins showed, in 1941, that castration (removal of the testicles) slowed progression of prostate cancer, physicians have assumed it was the resulting lack of testosterone that slowed the cancer, and ever since have relied on suppression of testosterone in their treatment of the disease. However, the testosterone suppression benefit only lasts two to three years, and then the prostate cancer progresses to an androgen (male hormone) insensitive state and continues to spread. Despite this, metastatic prostate cancer patients are treated with androgen blockade through castration (orchiectomy) and/or hormone-suppressing drugs.

Dr. Lee's Healthy Prostate Programme

1 **Diet should avoid sugars**, refined starches, and other glycemic (insulin raising) foods as well as high oestrogen food such as feedlot-raised meat and milk.

2 **Avoid xenooestrogens** such as pesticides and some plastics.

3 **Maintain a good intake of antioxidants**. It is known that chronic inflammation may be potentially carcinogenic. It is wise, therefore, to maintain one's intake of antioxidants such as vitamin C, selenium, and the fat soluble anti-oxidant vitamins, A, E, D, and K.

4 **If you are over 50, monitor saliva hormone levels** of progesterone and testosterone.

5 **Supplement progesterone and testosterone** by transdermal cream to maintain saliva levels consistent with that of healthy mature males. When supplemented in this manner, the doses required are quite small: I recommend 8 to 10 mg per day of progesterone and 1 to 2 mg per day of testosterone.

6 From my clinical experience, it would not surprise me that **exercise and an active sex life** are also protective factors against prostate cancer.

I remember reading studies done 30 to 40 years ago showing that testosterone supplementation prevented survival of prostate cancer cells transplanted to test mammals. In more recent (as yet unpublished) studies it has been shown that in a prostate cancer cell culture, testosterone kills the cancer cells. A 1996 study showed that in mice, testosterone will shrink human prostate tumours.[1]

Tracking the culprit

Why does prostate cancer occur so often in aging men? Consider the changes in testicular hormone production as men age:

1 Testosterone leves fall;

2 More testosterone is changed (by 5 alpha-reductase enzyme) to dihydrotestosterone (DHT), stimulating prostate growth;

3 Progesterone levels fall. Progesterone is vital to good health in men. It is the primary precursor of our adrenal cortical hormones and testosterone. Men synthesise progesterone in smaller amounts than women do but it is still vital. Since progesterone is a potent inhibitor of 5-alpha-reductase, the decline of progesterone in aging males plays a role in increasing the conversion rate of testosterone to DHT.

4   Oestradiol (an oestrogen) effect increases. Testosterone is a direct antagonist of oestradiol. Both the fall in testosterone and the shift from testosterone to DHT allows increased effect of oestradiol. Male oestradiol levels are equivalent to or greater than those of postmenopausal females, but normally oestradiol's effects are suppressed (antagonised) by the male's greater production of testosterone. Perhaps oestradiol is also the culprit (along with DHT) in prostate growth.

Getting down to the gene level

Embryology teaches us that the prostate is the male equivalent of the female uterus. The two organs differentiate from the same embryonic cells and they share many of the same genes such as the oncogene, Bcl-2, and the cancer-protector gene, p53. It is not surprising then that the hormonal relationships in endometrial cancer will be the same in prostate cancer; that is both are very sensitive to the harmful effects of unopposed oestrogen and are protected by progesterone. T. S. Wiley and Bent Formby, Ph.D. have done test tube studies that verify this relationship, but human studies still need to be done.

The course of prostate cancer growth, like breast cancer growth, is not due to a linear progression of cancer cells multiplying from one rogue cell; it is due to the continued presence of an underlying metabolic imbalance. The underlying metabolic imbalance in all hormone-dependent cancers is oestrogen dominance. Prevent the oestrogen dominance and you will prevent the cancer. If the cancer is already underway, correcting the oestrogen dominance will slow the cancer growth and prolong life. The benefit of castration in prostate cancer stemmed from oestradiol reduction, not testosterone reduction. Given the choice, I would choose testosterone and progesterone supplementation over castration.

15

How to use natural progesterone

FIRST, WE MUST BE CLEAR about what is meant by natural progesterone. There are, of course, a large number of plants containing progesterone-like compounds just as a large number of plants contain oestrogen-like compounds. Throughout this book, I have tried to be consistent in referring to these 'natural' oestrogen-like compounds as 'oestrogenic' substances. There is no specific hormone named 'oestrogen'; oestrogen is a class name and there are 20 or so members of this class made by the human body; the major ones being oestrone, oestradiol, and oestriol. In the case of proges-terone, there is but one pro-gestational hormone made by the human body and its name is progesterone. Its molecular configuration is pictured in Figure 1 in Chapter 2. *That* is what is meant by natural progesterone.

From what source does the natural progesterone used in various treatment forms come? Early in the course of progesterone research history, proges-terone was obtained from sows' corpora lutea. This was expensive and of low yield. A better source is the human placenta. The placenta is a veritable prog-esterone factory, making 300-400 mg per day during the last trimester of pregnancy. At childbirth, placentas can be quick-frozen and sent to a phar-maceutical firm for extraction of the progesterone they contain. Even more economical is the use of progesterone-like plant sterols, named saponins. Upon hydrolyzation, saponins are converted to sapogenins, of which two (sarsasapogenin and diosgenin) are the main source for the derivation of natural progesterone for medical use.

Through the wonders of modern chemistry, it is possible to synthesize progesterone from air, coal, and water but starting from the ready-made sapogenins from plants is by far the more efficient and productive way to go. From them, pure U.S.P. grade progesterone can be produced inexpensively and in great quantity.

Ironically, the majority of progesterone produced is bought by other phar-maceutical firms for further synthesis to 'un-natural' progesterone-like compounds, termed progestins, for use in their patent(ed) medicines. (See

Chapter 3.) Some progestins are synthesized from the male hormone, testosterone, such as might be obtained from horse urine, as the hormone, oestrone, is for Premarin (from pregnant mares).

The importance of understanding this derivation of progesterone from plant saponins is two-fold. One, in cultures wherein fresh saponin-rich plants such as yams constitute a major portion of the diet, some progesterone-like effects are derived from them. The July 1992 *National Geographic* contained a report of life on the Trobriand Islands (a small island group off S.E. New Guinea) and the people who are generally slim and happy, enjoy wonderful health (except for tuberculosis, leprosy, and malaria), have a vigorous sexual life and (strangely, to the authors) fewer children than might be expected, and whose diet is dedicated to the yam, other vegetables, and fish. The yam, in fact, is a Trobriand totem signifying good health and good life. Trobriand islanders regard their life as idyllic, as do the occasional visitors. The November 1992 *National Geographic* contained several letters to the editor, explaining that yams contain the sterol, diosgenin, with progesterone-like effects which accounts for the Trobriander islanders idyllic life style and lower birth rate. Progesterone, after all, is the basis for all oral contraceptives. One writer reports that 'Organon, a leading producer of contraceptive pills, uses the diosgenin from Mexican yam roots as the raw material for its products.' Yet, more than a few US physicians have no idea that their progestins are made from yams.

Second, products that list yam extract among their ingredients may or may not include the saponin-rich portion of yam root; and they may or may not include actual U.S.P. grade progesterone derived from yam (or a number of other plant sources) which is widely available. The reason for this confusion will be difficult for readers not familiar with the US to understand.

The reason stems not from a deliberate deception on the part of the product producers but from our set of poorly worded laws regulating drugs as distinguished from herbs, foods, drinks, confections, and condiments, apparently operating under the delusion that the biochemical effects from such-like are somehow different than those from 'drugs'. To sell 'drugs', you see, requires a licence and a degree of some kind, whereas just about anybody can sell foods and herbs.

As if this confusion were not bad enough, the US FDA (Federal Drug Administration) has occasional fits of over-zealous interpretation of the laws and attacks purveyors of teas and vitamins and what-not with costly legal suits and little comprehension of the facts of the matter. Thus the contrivance of benign labelling. Admittedly not a good thing, but I think it is helpful to understand the basis of the present confusion.

My reason for going into all this is that I am about to tell you how I use a progesterone product to treat various conditions and I am not all that familiar with all the progesterone products now on the market. I became interested in this in 1978 when I heard Professor Ray Peat, Ph.D., of Blake College, Eugene, Oregon, talk about the various attributes of progesterone. It was from him that I learned of a certain skin cream, called 'Cielo', and sold as a skin moisturizer (and it certainly is), which contained, among its other ingredients, natural progesterone. Later, when confronted with osteoporotic patients who could not use oestrogen because of history of uterine or breast cancer, or diabetes, or vascular disorders, etc., I chose to recommend this cream, hoping it would do something for their bones. And, to my considerable surprise, it did; their bone mineral density tests showed progressive improvement! Not knowing what dose to give, I used serial BMD tests to adjust dosage so that improvement occurred. It did not matter to me what dose of progesterone was in the cream; what mattered was that (1) it was safe to use, and (2) the right dose is the one that works.

Over the years since then, other companies have developed other products containing progesterone, and some use yam extract or other extract purported to simulate progesterone's effects. I recommend only those products that contain progesterone. From following the literature, I know that Dr. Joel T. Hargrove, of Vanderbilt University Medical Centre, uses progesterone in capsule form; and Dr. Katherine Dalton, of London, England, uses progesterone in rectal suppositories.

There are now a large number of companies marketing progesterone cream. I prefer those that contain 450-500 mg of progesterone per ounce (900-1000 mg per 2-oz container). I find them easy to dose. My goal is to restore normal physiologic levels of progesterone to balance oestrogen in women deficient in progesterone. This is accomplished most often by using 12-15 mg of progesterone per day. In postmenopausal women, 12-15 mg per day for 24-25 days is approximately 300 mg/month, or one-third of a 2-oz jar or container each month.

I am not a fan of other delivery systems. Sublingual drops are quickly absorbed but the duration of saliva levels from them is only two hours or so. Vaginal and rectal doses are similar. Oral doses are inefficient and result in liver metabolites, some of which can lead to lethargy. Transdermal absorption is superior, in my opinion, because absorption is excellent and saliva testing shows smooth levels lasting about 12 hours. Thus, twice-daily doses of progesterone cream supply 24 hours of normal physiologic levels which more closely match the body's needs.

Testing for progesterone

The saliva hormone assay

Much confusion has arisen with regard to the difference between concentrations of hormones in blood serum (or plasma) on the one hand, and in saliva on the other.

After all, if progesterone protects against breast cancer, it seems only logical to recommend that any woman with low progesterone levels should use a progesterone supplement.

But the reason why many doctors resist this idea is that, despite abundant proof, they do not understand *why* transdermal progesterone is absorbed well enough to provide physiologic levels. They apparently do not realise that progesterone is the most fat-loving (lipophilic) of all steroids, and is therefore not usually present in serum (which is the watery part of blood) unless it is protein-bound. This leads to serious misunderstandings, and a misreading of test results.

'Blood tests' for progesterone refer to the concentration of progesterone in serum or plasma. Plasma is the watery, non-cellular portion of the blood from which cellular components such as red blood cells and white blood cells are excluded. (Serum is essentially the same as plasma except that fibrinogen has been removed. For the purposes of this discussion serum and plasma are interchangeable, and I will refer to them as serum.)

Sex hormones such as progesterone, oestrogen and testosterone are fat-soluble steroids similar to cholesterol.

The ovary-produced progesterone found in serum has been made water-soluble by being bound to special proteins: as they circulate through the liver, they are separated from their protein binding and are metabolised for excretion in bile. In the case of progesterone, not only is 92-98% of the hormone in serum (or plasma) protein-bound, but *the protein-bound hormone is not bioavailable*. Only 2-5% of serum progesterone is 'free' or non-protein-bound. Thus progesterone measured by serum levels is mostly a measure of progesterone that is not going to be used by the body. A serum test serves to compare one woman's progesterone production to that of another woman, or to test how much progesterone is being made by a woman's ovaries.

When progesterone is given intravenously, 80% of it is taken up by red blood cell membranes that are fatty in nature and therefore available to fat-soluble progesterone molecules. Less than 20% will be found in serum. It is obvious that serum measures would not detect the great majority of the progesterone added to whole blood.

Absorption of transdermal progesterone

Progesterone is a highly lipophilic (fat loving) molecule that is well absorbed through skin into the underlying fat layer and enters the blood stream slowly by riding on the fatty membranes of red blood cells in capillaries passing through the fat. Since it is not protein-bound, essentially all of it is bioavailable to progesterone receptors is target tissues throughout the body. Very little of it would be found by serum or plasma testing.

Yet many doctors continue to question the skin absorption of progesterone. A recent example is a report in *The Lancet* (April 25, 1998, pp1255-6) stating that serum levels did not reflect a substantial rise of progesterone after topical application in postmenopausal women. This report is being used to argue that progesterone is not well absorbed through the skin from the application of Pro-Gest or similar creams.

This implication is erroneous. It simply means that the authors did not understand the significant difference between the levels of progesterone measured in serum and in saliva. Some doctors even imply that saliva testing is relatively unknown and its reliability unproved: an odd statement, since researchers have been using saliva testing for years and a number of laboratories offer routine saliva hormone testing.

A researcher using serum or plasma tests for measuring transdermally absorbed progesterone is testing the wrong portion of the blood. Saliva hormone assay, *not* a blood (i.e. serum or plasma) test, is the proper test for measuring non-protein-bound progesterone: progesterone in the blood filters through the saliva glands, so the saliva progesterone level is an accurate reflection of bioavailable blood progesterone levels in the body. It is also very stable, easily obtained, and proper saliva tests are very accurate.

Using the saliva hormone assay to determine progesterone dosage

The goal of progesterone supplementation is to restore natural physiologic levels of bioavailable progesterone. Progesterone/oestrogen balance is the key. When sufficient numbers of normally ovulating women are tested by saliva hormone assay, the typical range of progesterone is found to be 0.3 to 0.5

ng/ml. Under usual circumstances, there should be no reason to exceed that range.

In my experience the topical dose required to achieve a saliva level of 0.5 ng/ml is commonly only 12 to 15 mg per day. For creams containing 900 to 1000 mg per 2-oz container, 12-15 mg a day for 24 days would use up only about one-third of the container. Larger doses are often used initially to 'catch up' on the existing progesterone deficiency state, but the maintenance dose will usually be around 15 mg a day. Since considerable variation in progesterone is well tolerated, a modest elevation of saliva levels to 0.8 to 1.5 ng/ml is acceptable.

For the many doctors who are confused about hormone balance, wider use of saliva hormone assays would help their understanding of their patients' problems. It is an ongoing tragedy that the use and benefits of progesterone are so little understood by conventional physicians.

Progesterone treatment recommendations: General considerations

A. Transdermal absorption

It is well known that all the gonadal hormones, being small, fat-soluble molecules, are well absorbed through the skin; better, in fact, than when given orally. Oestradiol, for instance, given as a transdermal patch containing 0.05 mg applied twice weekly is equivalent to oral doses of 1 mg daily. That is, 0.1 mg transdermally = 7 mg orally, or 70 times more efficient, the difference being the first-pass loss through the liver of oral doses. Similar efficiency occurs with testosterone and progesterone.

B. Distribution throughout the body

In applying progesterone-containing cream, I recommend using the largest possible areas of relatively thin skin, rotating among various skin sites daily for maximum absorption. Skin sites recommended are the inner aspects of the arms and thighs, the face and neck, the upper chest, and the abdomen. In dermal transport, progesterone is first absorbed into the subcutaneous fat layer and then passively diffused throughout the body via blood circulation. Initially, in progesterone-deficient patients, much of the progesterone is absorbed into body fat. With continued use, fat levels of progesterone reach an equilibrium such that successive doses of progesterone result in increased blood levels and stronger physiological effects. Thus, it is wise to tell women that progesterone applications may require two to three months of use before maximum benefits are experienced.

When produced by the corpus luteum, progesterone is embedded in a protein envelope, cortisol binding globulin (CBG), for solubility in plasma, with only 2-10% of progesterone in the free (unbound) state. Similarly, oestrogen is embedded in sex hormone binding globulin (SHBG) for transport in plasma; and cholesterol is circulated enveloped in various lipo-proteins. It is not presently known whether progesterone absorbed transdermally or orally acquires a CBG carrier envelope or whether it binds temporarily to fat soluble components of cell membranes (such as, of red blood cells) for transport through blood circulation. Thus, plasma progesterone levels may not accurately measure the total progesterone available. Dosage adequacy is determined ultimately by the effects produced. (See 'Progesterone dosage' below.)

In postmenopausal women concomitantly using oestrogen supplements, the initial effect of progesterone is to sensitize oestrogen receptors, leading to heightened oestrogen effects such as breast swelling and tenderness, fluid retention, or even the appearance of scant vaginal bleeding. Therefore, I generally advise such women to reduce their oestrogen dose by one-half when starting on progesterone.

Later, after 3-4 months of progesterone use, many women can reduce their oestrogen dose further or eventually discontinue it, using adequacy of vaginal secretions as their guide.

During the perimenopausal phase, when women are experiencing changing patterns of menstruation, including missed menses, the addition of natural progesterone may temporarily bring a return to normal monthly menses. This temporary heightened sensitivity of oestrogen receptors may lead the woman (and her doctor) to conclude that progesterone *caused* the menses, whereas, in fact, the normal oestrogen caused the endometrial proliferation and the quitting of the progesterone each month (see 'Dosage cycling' below), allowed the shedding of whatever proliferative endometrium had developed. This is a normal state of affairs and not a cause for alarm.

C. Dosage cycling

Continued exposure of hormone signals (or other receptor signals such as sound or light) leads eventually to reduced receptor sensitivity. Our receptors 'tune down' their sensitivity to prolonged exposure by the receptor stimulator. This is obvious in the case of sound or light. A sufficient period of quiet will bring about renewed sensitivity to sound just as a period of darkness will allow increased sensitivity to dim light, so-called 'dark adaptation'. The same is true of transdermal nitroglycerin, for instance. If nitroglycerine patches or ointment are used continuously, its effect on coronary artery relaxation will diminish; occasional periods of non-use will restore its effectiveness. And the same is true of the hormones. Recall that, during regular monthly menstruation, there occurs a week or so each month of low hormone levels.

Thus, I recommend that progesterone be cycled monthly. In postmenopausal women, progesterone may be used 24-26 days of the month and then discontinued until the next month. A period of at least 4-5 days should be hormone free. In perimenopausal patients, I recommend timing the progesterone use to approximate normal corpus luteal production of progesterone, i.e. from day 12 to day 26 of the menstrual cycle. On occasion, this may be difficult to do with precision if menses are occurring irregularly. If, after using progesterone for a week or so and some spotting occurs, I usually recommend that the progesterone be halted for 12 days and then started anew.

D. Progesterone dosage

Though it is known that normal corpus luteum progesterone production may reach 20-25 mg per day, it is also true that wide individual variability is the rule. The same is probably also true of one's efficiency in transdermal absorption. Further, since oestrogen and progesterone have many mutual antagonistic effects, prevailing oestrogen levels will effect the results of a given dose of progesterone. Third, the progesterone dose must be related to the effect one wishes to promote.

In PMS, the dose must be high to counter the effects of prevailing, previously unopposed, oestrogen. The dose is determined essentially by trial and error. The same is true in the perimenopausal state. After menopause, when oestrogen levels are low and the desired effect is new bone formation, effective progesterone doses may be considerably lower than those needed for PMS. In treating postmenopausal osteoporosis, serial BMD testing can be used to determine progesterone dose. Thus, clinical judgment by both the patient and her doctor is desirable for the most effective use of supplemental natural progesterone. Because of the great safety of natural progesterone, considerable latitude is allowed.

E. When a woman is also on a progestin

When a woman on progestins wishes to switch to natural progesterone, several considerations should be kept in mind. First, both compete for receptor sites. The benefits of natural progesterone will be seriously reduced by the presence of the progestin. Second, plasma progesterone levels will not reach maximum levels until the 2nd or 3rd month of use, as described in B above. I recommend simply stopping progestin use when starting natural progesterone.

F. When a woman is on thyroid medication

Cellular utilization of thyroid hormone is impeded by oestrogen and promoted by progesterone. Thus, a woman with oestrogen dominance, whether endogenous or by supplement use, may experience symptoms of hypothyroidism.

Despite normal T-3 and T-4 serum levels, the thyroid stimulating hormone (TSH) level may indeed be elevated, indicating a need for thyroid supplements. When such a patient on thyroid medication receives natural progesterone supplementation, cellular utilization of thyroid hormone becomes more efficient again. If not checked by repeat TSH testing, it is likely that continued use of thyroid medication will result in the patient becoming hyperthyroid. The lessons here are (1) that T-3 and T-4 levels are not as reliable as TSH level for determining need for thyroid supplementation, and (2) that natural progesterone facilitates enhanced efficiency of cellular utilization of thyroid hormone, a factor that should be monitored when adding progesterone therapy in people using thyroid medication.

Osteoporosis prevention and/or treatment

1. Postmenopausal patients

Progesterone is a vital link in a chain of multiple factors which, together, are necessary for good bone building. This chain includes proper diet, a few nutrient supplements, exercise, avoidance of cigarette smoking, and hormones. One or another of the factors, if missing, will prevent the chain from doing its work. A typical treatment program follows:

Diet Emphasize *fresh* vegetables, particularly broad leafy greens. Restrict or avoid 'sodas' and limit red meat to 3 or fewer times per week. Choose whole grains over refined flour. Limit alcohol use. Milk is not necessary and is not advisable for adults. Cheese, however, is OK.

Vitamin D 350-400 i.u. daily.

Vitamin C 2 grams daily in divided doses.

Betacarotene 15 mg/day (equivalent to 25,000 i.u. of vitamin A).

Zinc 15-30 mg/day.

Calcium Seek to obtain 800-1000 mg/day by diet and supplements.

Magnesium 300 - 800 mg/day supplement.

Oestrogen Contraindicated by history of breast or uterine cancer, clotting or vascular disorders, obesity, diabetes, fibrocystic breasts, and hyperlipidemia. If used, I would recommend low-dose conjugated oestrogen (e.g. Premarin 0.3 mg daily three weeks per month) rather than oestradiol. If available, oestriol (1-2 mg/day) would be preferred, being a safer oestrogen. If not needed for vaginal dryness or hot flushes, it need not be used, depending on the results of serial BMD tests.

Progesterone I usually recommend transdermal application (e.g. Pro-Gest or equivalent cream) sufficient to use up 1 ounce of the cream per month, being applied daily for 24-26 days per month in postmenopausal women. In premenopausal women, cream is applied from day 12 to day 26 of the menstrual month, using one-third of a 2-oz container, planning to stop a day or so before the expected period. If oestrogen is being used for menpausal women, both hormones should be discontinued during the same 4-6 days each month. When repeat BMD testing reveals increasing bone density, progesterone dose may be reduced to one-third of a 2-oz container per month.

Exercise I recommend vigorous exercise for 20 minutes daily or ½ hour at least 3 times per week.

No cigarettes. Report any occurrence of vaginal bleeding.

Dosing with transdermal progesterone cream

In advising patients on progesterone dosage, I prefer to have them think in terms of monthly dose, rather than a daily dose. It is my experience that, if patients are asked to use ¼ or ½ tsp. of cream daily, the monthly totals are quite variable. For instance, one patient may report that she may use up 2 ounces or more of the cream each month using ½ tsp. daily, whereas another patient will report that her 2-oz jar lasts two or more months using supposedly the same daily dose. On the other hand, when the patient is advised to use up the 1-oz portion over the course of a month, she quickly learns what size 'gob' to use daily or twice a day to accomplish this monthly dose in the allotted time period, whether it be two weeks or three. Later, if the patient's monthly dose is reduced to one-third of a 2-oz container, I instruct her to use a spoon to transfer the contents of a 2-oz jar into three smaller jars, with each to be used over the course of a month.

2. Perimenopausal patients

As is often the case, a premenopausal woman may find on BMD testing that she is already losing bone mass (see Chapter 9). In such cases, I recommend the same general program listed above but using the transdermal natural progesterone cream in such a way as to approximate normal function of the corpus luteum, i.e., applying the cream from day 12 to day 26 of the menstrual month. Again, I would ask the patient to use up a 2-oz jar of Pro-Gest cream during this 2-week time period. Later, as BMD tests rise to indicate new bone formation, I would try decreasing the cream to 1 oz monthly and follow the results with serial BMD tests at 6-month or yearly intervals. Oestrogen would not be used in these cases.

Note: On using BMD tests

Since trabecular bone has a more rapid turnover time, I have found that lumbar vertebra are excellent for following the course of osteoporosis treatment results. The changes occur there sooner than they can be observed or measured in denser cortical bone. Further, being relatively large and uniform, the test results are generally more consistently accurate. I recognize that the hip fracture risk is more clinically important but it is essential to establish that the treatment plan is, in truth, effective in promoting osteoporosis reversal. When this is found, patient compliance is greatly enhanced. It should be recalled that, like hypertension, osteoporosis is a silent disorder (until catastrophe occurs) and the patient should have the opportunity to monitor treatment progress just as blood pressure readings are necessary to monitor hypertension treatment.

Further, I recommend use of dual photon absorptiometry (DPA) or dual energy X-ray absorptiometry (DEXA) rather than the quantified CT (QCT) test because (1) equivalent accuracy and sensitivity, (2) DPA and DEXA use much less radiation exposure than QCT, and (3) both are less costly than QCT. When performing serial testing, it should be remembered that the different techniques give slightly different results and, therefore, comparisons of test results using different techniques are not as good as using the same technique throughout. Further, it is wise to use the same equipment in the same testing facility, if possible. (See Chapter 11 for a more detailed consideration of BMD testing.)

Fibrocystic breasts

Fibrocystic breasts are caused by oestrogen dominance. It is the experience of my patients that restoring hormone balance with natural progesterone usually results in prompt clearing of the problem. The typical patient presents with a history of repeated episodes of painful, cystic breasts, commonly worse during the week or so before menses and clearing after menses; and she already knows to avoid caffeine (methyl xanthine) from coffee, tea, colas and chocolate, and has tried vitamin E without sufficient relief. Often the patient reports having undergone repeated needle drainage and/or biopsies and is fearful of breast cancer. When natural progesterone is used (e.g., a 2-oz jar of Pro-Gest cream) during the two weeks before menses, fibrocystic breasts revert to normal within 2-3 months. Later, the patient may find that application of only one ounce of the cream during this time interval each month will prevent recurrence.

Vignette #1. I recall being asked on one occasion (during the early eighties when I was first discovering for myself the multiple benefits of natural progesterone) to be a member of a physicians' panel discussing fibrocystic breast 'disease' (as it was called in those days) at a national health symposium in San Francisco. I felt honoured to be so invited and initially gave no thought to the fact that the meeting was sponsored by a consortium of pharmaceutical companies. In the course of the panel discussion, the moderator asked me to describe the typical patient with fibrocystic breasts. He then asked me what I would do if all the typical treatments (diet, avoiding methyl xanthines, vitamin E, etc.) failed to relieve the problem. I, of course, proceeded to tell the panel and the audience of the success that comes from using natural progesterone. With that, the moderator became quite flustered, turned red in the face, and started perspiring profusely. It turns out he had wanted to introduce Danazol, the synthetic, androgenic anti-oestrogen steroid new at the time, and all the questions from other panel members and the audience concerned natural progesterone and how to obtain it. Our panel had been designed to illustrate the failure of conventional treatment for fibro-cystic breasts and to advertize the new drug. The moderator was clearly discomfited by the news about natural progesterone and my presentation of it. I was never invited to be a panel member again.

Vignette #2. On another occasion, I had consulted with an elderly lady about using natural progesterone for osteoporosis. In the course of our conversation, she asked about fibrocystic breasts. After doing so, I expressed surprise that she would be bothered by that problem because she had not used oestrogen; at which point she said she planned to relay the information to her daughter in Arizona who was scheduled for bilateral mastectomies due to her severe fibrocystic breast problem. Six weeks later, after two cycles of natural progesterone, the daughter called me from Arizona and related that, much to her surgeon's surprise, the breast problem had cleared completely and surgery had been cancelled.

Vignette #3. A feisty lady in her late seventies consulted with me about her advanced osteoporosis, having had several spinal compression fractures. She had previously avoided hormone therapy because of a long history of fibrocystic breasts prior to menopause. With natural progesterone applications, her BMD rose gratifyingly, her back pains disappeared, and she resumed normal activities such as hiking, boating, gardening, etc. Several years later, after I retired from active practice, she came under the care of a new doctor who convinced her that she should abandon progesterone and use oestrogen instead. On reluctantly doing so, she soon developed painful fibrocystic breasts and her new doctor was now recommending bilateral mastectomy to avoid possible breast cancer. Upset at this turn of events, she called me to ask how she should respond to the doctor's advice. I told her to (1) immediately discontinue the oestrogen and return to the progesterone that had done so well for her bones and had kept her breasts free of cysts, (2) obtain a mammogram to relieve her worry about breast cancer, and (3) tell the doctor he should have a bilateral orchiectomy to avoid possible prostate cancer. At this, she laughed heartily and promised to follow my advice completely. Back on natural progesterone, she has remained healthy and active to this date. I don't know if her doctor learned anything from the experience.

Premenstrual syndrome (PMS)

As described in Chapter 10, PMS is a complex, multi-factorial syndrome. Being able to provide reliable relief of PMS symptoms will result in the most appreciative of patients. Natural progesterone, if given in sufficient doses, will accomplish this in a remarkable majority of cases. The fact that it does not do so in *all* cases merely implies that the syndrome may result from other factors also.

My recommendation for PMS, especially for those with all the hallmarks of oestrogen dominance (e.g. breast swelling and premenstrual fluid retention), is to use a 1-oz portion of Pro-Gest in a ten-day period, ending just before expected menses. With experience, many patients discover that the progesterone dose can be applied in a manner to produce a crescendo effect in the 4-5 days just prior to menses. In fact, some prefer to add sublingual progesterone drops during the last 4-5 days in addition to the transdermal cream. Other patients find that additional cream may be applied several times a day depending on their symptoms. As with other conditions discussed, the right dose of progesterone is the dose that works.

If proof of progesterone deficiency is desired, it is possible to test the plasma progesterone level 4-7 days after supposed ovulation time. A low level at that time confirms lack of corpora luteal progesterone production and the probable need of progesterone supplementation.

The major contribution of natural progesterone does not preclude proper attention to other contributing factors such as diet, calcium and/or magnesium supplements, vitamin B6, vitamin E, relaxation techniques and good exercise. Dietary factors include avoidance of sugar, refined carbohydrates, and refined fats, choosing instead plenty of fresh vegetables of all sorts, and ensuring a good intake of the essential fatty acids as from Primrose oil, Flaxseed oil, or Blackcurrant oil. There are several herbal remedies that also have reportedly been found effective: these include vitex agnus castus, yellow dock, burdock root, wild yam root, licorice root, fo-ti, pau d'arco, dong quai, astragalus, ginger, oatstraw, comfrey, nettle, raspberry leaf, squawvine, motherwort, horsetail, and red clover. As I do not claim to be expert in these herbal matters, I would recommend consulting with a herbal expert regarding their use.

When using a saliva assay, saliva progesterone levels serveral times higher than 0.5 ng/ml are justified in situations where stress is a factor, as is often true in the case of PMS. Stress increases cortisol production. Cortisol blockades some progesterone receptors and thereby prevents progesterone function. To compete with this blockade, topical progesterone in the range of 30 to 40 mg a day is sometimes initially required to achieve a beneficial effect.

Ovarian cysts

Ovarian cysts refer to follicle cysts or corpus luteum cysts and represent a failure of normal follicle development and ovulation, leaving the corpus luteum in a condition such that subsequent monthly FSH, LH and oestrogen surges result in an enlarging benign cyst. Follicle cysts result in a persistent proliferative endometrium (due to absence of progesterone production); and corpus luteum cysts result in a prolonged secretory phase (due to continuing progesterone production). Natural progesterone, given from day 5 to day 26 of the menstrual month for 2-3 cycles, will almost routinely cause the cyst to disappear by suppressing normal FSH, LH and oestrogen production, giving the ovary time to heal. Here again, the progesterone in a 1-oz portion of trans-dermal Pro-Gest cream applied monthly is usually sufficient. Progress can be monitored by pelvic exam or by sonograms. Ovarian cysts are more common at age 30+, when follicle depletion is advanced.

Uterine fibroids

Uterine fibroids are another example of oestrogen dominance secondary to anovulatory cycles and consequent progesterone deficiency. They generally occur in the 8-10 years before menopause. If sufficient natural progesterone is supplemented from day 12 to day 26 of the menstrual cycle, further growth of fibroids is usually prevented (and often the fibroids regress). After menopause, oestrogen levels become low and fibroids eventually atrophy. Progesterone dosage can be determined by results shown by serial pelvic sono-gram tests every 3-4 months.

Cervical erosions and/or dysplasia

These are tissue-specific reactions to folic acid deficiency and, possibly, hormone imbalance. When folic acid (a B vitamin) is given in doses of 3-5 mg per day along with vitamin B6 (50 mg/day) and magnesium (300 mg/day), recovery usually takes place in 1-2 cycles. Progress can be followed by serial Pap smears. If recovery is delayed, intravaginal progesterone cream or intravaginal oestriol applied daily during the month between menses should restore normal cervical epithelium. Specific dosage is not known with preci-sion, but $1/4$ tsp. of the Pro-Gest cream inserted intravaginally each day is found to be successful.

Summary

Natural progesterone is remarkably effective, safe, and relatively inexpensive therapy for a wide range of female disorders resulting from oestrogen domi-nance. A user-friendly technique of using transdermal progesterone cream has been presented here.

16

Progesterone and the medical-industrial complex

'IF NATURAL PROGESTERONE is so wonderful, why isn't it used by my doctor?' This is the question I am most frequently asked. My answer is that it is not favoured by the medical-industrial complex. The reasons for my answer derive not from a systematic study of the problem but from personal experience of over thirty years of active clinical practice and observing the various ways, some subtle and some not so subtle, medical practice is influenced.

The medical-industrial complex refers to the close-knit association of organized medicine with pharmaceutical manufacturers and governmental medical regulatory agencies. The connections between these groups is, of course, a web of money, power, and prestige. The system taken together is neither necessarily corrupt nor evil but, like any human agency, is subject to the frailties and faults of humankind. Selling medical drugs is *very big* business. Medical research is dependent on the $billions of grants from the National Institutes of Health (NIH) and the private pharmaceutical industry. The two are closely interlocked; managers in one tend to have come from success in the other with many examples of interchangeable personnel.

Any given pharmaceutical company, like any private enterprise, must make a profit to stay alive. Profit comes from sales of patent medicines. The system is not interested in natural (non-patentable) medicines, regardless of their potential health benefits. Thus, the flow of research funding does not extend to products which can not be patented. Experts in research, therefore, tend to have experience only with patented drugs and little or none with natural products or non-patentable procedures. When an NIH or industry-supported academic 'expert' speaks on the subject of a natural product or, say, acupuncture, you can be sure that he has had very little, if any, experience using it; or, if he speaks from the literature, you can be sure it is the literature of the medical-industrial establishment. The recent widely-advertised open-mindedness of the NIH to alternative therapies is not sufficiently funded to more than lightly touch on a few items of the wide field that actually exists.

Few people know that the definition of malpractice hinges on whether or not the practice is common among one's medical peers and has little (usually nothing) to do with whether the practice is beneficial or not. A doctor willing to study, to learn the ins and outs of an alternative medical therapy, and to put what he has learned into practice in helping patients is potentially exposing himself to serious charges of malpractice. And he can expect no help from organized medicine. Truth be known, medicine today is very disorganized and what passes as 'organized medicine' is merely a handmaiden to the powers of health agencies and the pharmaceutical industry. The great majority of academic physicians, for instance, do not bother to belong to the AMA. Why should they, when all money and career advances come from the mercy of the funding agencies?

But what has all this to do with natural progesterone? The answer is quite simple, really. Ample medical research regarding progesterone was carried on in the 1940s through the 1960s, and amply reported in mainline, recognized medical literature. Since the early 1970s, however, medical research has become much more expensive and the grants subsidizing progesterone (or any unpatentable medicine or treatment technique) research have dried up and been blown away by the contemporary trade winds of synthetic drugs, particularly the progestins. The potential market for patentable progestins is vast — contraceptive pills, irregular menses, osteoporosis, prevention of endometrial cancer — literally every woman through every age from puberty on is a target for a sale. Do you think the prevailing powers wish to see this lucrative market be left to an over-the-counter natural product not in the hands of physician prescribers and not controlled by the pharmaceutical industry?

Licensed doctors are easy to control. All practising US physicians must accumulate a given number of hours of 'continuing medical education' or CME. Sounds like a good idea, doesn't it? But where do they acquire their CME credits? From authorized CME seminars, that's where. And who authorizes which seminar for CME credits? Organized medicine, that's who. And who sponsors and who provides the speakers for CME-credited seminars? The pharmaceutical industry and its grant-funded corps of academic researchers, that's who. US physicians are the captive audience for pharmaceutical advertising. They learn which drugs to prescribe. They do not learn of alternative and perhaps better ways of treating illness. If a doctor were to seek this information for himself, he finds himself outside the realm and benevolence of his professional guild. Further, he is reluctant to be perceived as practising in a manner different than his peers not only because of his fraternal associations with them but also because of the threat of malpractice charges, however unfounded.

Thus, when he hears of the uses of natural progesterone, he wonders why none of his associates knows about it. If it is not commonly known, it must in some way be false and/or unapproved. Having given lectures on the role and medical uses of natural progesterone, I have observed numerous instances wherein perfectly fine physicians will inquire about obtaining the product for use by their wives or mother-in-law but not for their patients. What can account for such behaviour by professionals? I suspect it is fear of alienation from the flock that is paramount in their minds.

How can this be changed? It will be changed when intelligent, motivated and assertive patients insist on this form of care. If progestins were the equivalent of natural progesterone in effect and safety, the argument would be moot. But progestins are not the equivalent of natural progesterone and never will be. It is extremely unlikely that man can synthesize a hormone better than the one Nature derived from aeons of natural selection.

Patients are aware that they can not leave their health care solely in the hands of the doctor. They must assume the responsibility for their own health. They must become knowledgeable and seek informed opinion from various sources. They know that the same medicine is not necessarily the best medicine for every individual. They want their medical advisors to join with them in a partnership for health; they will no longer put up with the present condescending child-parent relationship. Their empowerment must come through knowledge. This is the purpose of this book — to share the knowledge that I and others have accumulated over the past two to three decades of study, particularly as it pertains to progesterone, a natural hormone too remarkable to remain neglected.

Good health and long life to you all!

Afterword to the first edition

IF A FOREWORD, why not an afterword? This little book, eighteen months and four reprints after its first printing in the USA, is now in its first UK edition. During this brief time much has happened that deserves comment. I have received hundreds of letters and phone calls from readers and health providers concerning their experience and questions regarding natural progesterone, and several ground-breaking studies have been published to add considerable weight to the scientific evidence supporting the conclusions I had derived from my clinical experience with natural progesterone. This is my opportunity to bring readers up to date on matters of hormone replacement therapy.

One of the most interesting and relevant developments has been the matter of salivary hormone assays. Yes, all our steroid hormones are found in saliva and they can be accurately measured by radio immune assay (RIA) techniques. To understand the relevance of this, we must revisit serum hormone levels.

Steroid hormones (corticosteroids, DHEA, or the sex hormones) are fat-soluble compounds and generally not soluble in water, such as blood serum. To make them water-soluble and thus allow them to circulate in serum, the adrenal gland, ovary, and testes envelop the hormones they synthesize in a protein carrier or, in the case of DHEA, bind it to sulphate. Oestrogen hormones are enveloped in sex hormone binding globulin (SHBG) and progesterone is enveloped in cortisol binding globulin (CBG). The water-soluble protein-bound hormones, however, are not biologically active and thus are not a true measure of hormone activity. Only 1-10% of the serum levels of these hormones represent biologically active hormone. The hormone levels found in saliva, however, are measurements of only the active hormones. Thus, salivary hormone measurements are not only less expensive and more easily obtained but also are potentially more relevant.

Dr. Peter Ellison, from the Harvard anthropology department, has been particularly active in using salivary hormone levels in ecologic studies of human ovarian function among different populations around the world[1-3] and in tests of menstrual variation in the hormones of regularly cycling women.[4] From his work we learn that gonadal hormone levels of women in the Western or industrialized world are considerably different than hormone levels of women in the more agrarian (less industrialized) cultures of the so-called 'developing' world. Women of the industrialized world have considerably higher premenopausal levels of oestrogen and a greater fall in oestrogen levels at menopause. Dr. Ellison suggests that these differences may be the result of energetics, i.e. differences in dietary caloric intake relative to calorie requirements of physical labour. More abundant food intake correlates with earlier onset of menarche (age of starting menses) and with higher baseline levels of oestrogen. This finding may be a major factor in the more intense menopausal symptom experienced by women of industrialized societies.

Further, one of Dr. Ellison's studies involved a group of 18 women, average age 29, all with regular menstrual cycles.[4] He found that seven of these women showed no mid cycle rise in progesterone, indicating that they were not ovulating. This is merely another indication of the epidemic of anovulatory cycles and progesterone deficiency (and consequent oestrogen dominance) that occurs in premenopausal women in the US.

These salivary hormone assays are now becoming available. For example, Dr Zava at ZRT Laboratory (see 'Further information') now perform these tests routinely. Dr. Zava informs me that they are excellent tests to confirm that transdermal progesterone is well absorbed. Since natural progesterone in a skin cream is not enveloped in a protein coat it is not soluble in blood serum but yet shows up in good amounts within hours of applying it to the skin. Being fat-soluble it is probably carried in chylomicrons (minute fat droplets in blood) and on membranes of blood-borne cells such as red blood cells, and is available for tissues (including salivary glands) in the biologically active form. Interestingly, Dr. Zava found that the palms of the hands and the soles of feet are excellent skin sites for progesterone absorption.

A second important problem for many of my colleagues concerns the matter of protection against oestrogen-induced endometrial cancer. Doctors are aware that oestrogen replacement therapy (ORT) increases the risk of endometrial cancer and, thus, progestins are routinely added to decrease this risk. Lacking an approved reference showing that natural progesterone is perfectly capable of providing this same protection, they are reluctant to switch to natural progesterone for women receiving ORT. Fortunately, this problem is now resolved. A major report (the PEPI Trial) in the *JAMA* of 18 January 1995[5] found that both natural progesterone and medroxyproges- terone acetate (Provera) prevented adenomatous or atypical endometrial hyperplasia in women receiving ORT, while three years of ORT without a progestin or natural progesterone caused 34% of women to develop these potentially pre-cancerous changes.

A third factor concerns progesterone's effect on blood lipids. Here again, the PEPI study[5] sheds some light. Oestrogen supplementation results in improved total and HDL cholesterol levels. When medroxyprogesterone acetate is added, this benefit is markedly reduced. When natural progesterone was used, the benefits were maintained. Thus, the advantage goes to natural progesterone. Since many women continue to make adequate oestrogen after menopause and do very well on natural progesterone alone, it is unfortunate that this study did not include a cohort of women on progesterone alone. In my clinical experience, supplementation with natural progesterone alone improves one's lipid profile.

A fourth matter of some importance is the continued belief that oestrogen supplementation prevents and/or treats menopausal osteoporosis. Since the advent of dual photon and dual energy absorptiometry tests of bone mineral density, it has become obvious that osteoporosis starts long before menopause when oestrogen levels are still high and correlates more strongly with prog- esterone deficiency than with oestrogen deficiency. As I have described, menopausal oestrogen decline in industrialized women temporarily acceler- ates bone resorption. After 3-5 years, however, this accelerated bone loss settles back into the 'normal' bone loss rate of 1.5% per year whether or not the woman continues taking oestrogen supplements. New bone formation is a function of progesterone[6] and/or testosterone, and not of oestrogen. A major study of hip fracture risk factors in the *New England Journal of Medicine* of 23 March 19958 found that, for women 65 years or age or older, oestrogen supplementation at that time of life was not associated with prevention of hip fractures.[7] The typical woman using oestrogen had the same relative risk of hip fracture as one not using oestrogen. It is possible that the menopausal acceleration of bone loss will be decreased by oestrogen supplementation in women with signs of oestrogen deficiency. Such women will likely emerge from their perimenopausal years with better bones if oestrogen, along with natural progesterone, is also supplemented in small doses for 3-5 years around menopause. After this time in a woman's life, further supplementation of oestrogen will depend on such symptoms as vaginal atrophy or dryness, and not on the belief that it is needed for her bones. Progesterone, of course, can be continued throughout life since it maintains new bone formation.

From the above, the reader can be assured that the scientific evidence continues to add credibility to the important roles of natural progesterone. Transdermal absorption of physiologic dosages of natural progesterone is well established by the new salivary testing. Natural progesterone protects the uterus from undesirable oestrogen effects including oestrogen-induced adenomatous and atypical hyperplasia as well as the synthetic progestins, and provides an improved lipid profile. Further, there is strong evidence that osteoporotic hip fractures in women 65 years of age and older are not correlated with oestrogen supplementation at that age. The problem here is less due to accelerated bone resorption than to the lack of new bone formation; thus the need for progesterone.

I must conclude with a tribute to what I call the women's underground communication network, the vast informal woman-to-woman communication network that spreads hormone and health information with astonishing speed and extent around the world. An informational and health revolution is under way, thanks to the networking of intelligent, concerned women. If my little book has played a part in expanding the available knowledge of natural progesterone, I am proud to have been included in this process.

John R. Lee, MD
May 1995

Glossary

Definition of words of medical or biochemical nature that may be unfamiliar to the non-specialist reader.

adenomyosis islets of endometrial tissue within the muscular wall of the uterus leading to painful menstruation

amenorrhoea absence of menstruation

androgenic producing masculine characteristics

anovulatory suspension or cessation of ovulation

aromatization conversion of a cyclic organic compound to phenol-like form

blastoderm the early mass of cells produced by cleavage of a fertilized ovum

carcinogen any cancer-producing substance

catabolism the process by which living cells convert complex substances to simpler compounds, i.e., negative metabolism

catalyst any substance which affects the rate or velocity of a chemical reaction

chromosome the molecules that contain the genes (genomes), or hereditary factors, composed of DNA or RNA

coliform resembling E. coli, the common microbe in the colon

conjugated in biochemistry, one compound combined with another

corpus luteum small yellow glandular mass in the ovary formed by an ovarian follicle after ovulation (release of its egg [ovum])

corticosteroid hormones produced by the adrenal cortex

cytoplasm the watery protoplasm of a cell excluding the nucleus

de novo in biochemistry, refers to synthesis from basic components rather than from compounds synthesized in prior reactions

diuretic substances that increase urine production

DNA deoxyribonucleic acid, the basic component of chromosomes

dysmenorrhoea painful menstruation

ecologic related to the environment and life history of organisms, including man.

endocrine   refers to organs (glands) that secrete substances such as hormones

endogenous   developing or originating within the body

endometrium   the inner secretory lining of the uterus

enzyme   an organic compound, usually a protein, capable of catalytic action producing a change in some substrate for which it is often specific

exogenous   originating outside of the body

follicle   a very small excretory or secretory sac or gland, e.g., the ovarian follicle that produces the ovum

gamete   the ovum or the sperm, the union of which is necessary in sexual reproduction

genome   now used to connote gene, the hereditary units of chromosomes

gonadal   refers to the gamete-producing glands, i.e., ovaries and testes

gonadotropic   refers to hormones that affect or stimulate gonads

gram   unit of mass (weight), about 1/30th of an ounce

homeostasis   the body's ability to maintain a stable internal environment

hybridization   the process of producing a new of plant or animal from parents different in kind

hydrolyzed   refers to splitting a compound by the addition of water in which the hydroxyl group in incorporated in one fragment and the hydrogen atom in the other

hydroxylation   the addition of a hydroxyl radical (-OH) to a compound

hypermenorrhoea   excessive bleeding with menses

hypothalamus   neural nuclei of the limbic brain just above the pituitary which control visceral activities, water balance, sleep, and hormone production by the pituitary

hysterectomy   surgical removal of the uterus

libido   the sex drive

limbic brain   brain cortex below the corpus callosum and above the pituitary that contain neural nuclei controlling autonomic functions, homeostasis, emotional sensation and responses, and regulate immune responses

luteinizing   refers to maturation of ovarian follicles for ovulation after which the follicle become the corpus luteum producing progesterone

mastodynia   painful breasts

metabolism   the biochemical process of living organisms by which substances are produced and energy is made available to the organism

metrorrhagia   irregular menstruation

microgram   one-millionth (10^{-6}) of a gram

milligram   one-thousandth (10^{-3}) of a gram

mineralcorticoid   a corticoid particularly effective in causing sodium retention and potassium excretion

mitochondria   small organelles within the cytoplasm that are the site of converting sugar into energy; contains its own DNA

nanogram   one-billionth (10^{-9}) of a gram

oocytes   the cell that produces the ovum

oophorectomy   surgical removal of an ovary or ovaries

osteoblast   bone cell that forms new bone

osteoclast   bone cell that resorbs old bone

osteocyte   means bone cell; may become an osteoclast or an osteoblast

osteoid   the non-cellular collagenous matrix of bone

peptide   a class of low molecular weight compounds composed of several amino acids

perimenopausal   refers to the time preceding menopause when hormone changes are occurring

phyto-   denotes relationship to plants

premenopausal   prior to menopause

resorption   the loss or dissolving away of a substance

saprophyte   an organism that lives upon dead or decaying organic matter

steroid   group name for compounds based on cholesterol molecule, e.g., sex hormones and corticosteroids

sterol   compounds with single hydroxyl group (-OH) soluble in fats, widely found in plants and animals. Cholesterol is a sterol.

synovial   referring to the inner lining of joint spaces

thermogenic   capable of inducing a rise in temperature

trans-   combining form, referring to compounds that have been altered from their natural state

xeno-   combining form, meaning strange, or denoting relationship to foreign material

References

1. A history of progesterone

1 History of progesterone as described by Goodman & Gilman, *The Pharmacological Basis of Therapeutics*, sixth edition, 1980, Chapter 61, Estrogens and Progestins; pg.1420.

2 *Textbook of Clinical Chemistry*, Norbert W. Tietz, Ph.D., editor, W.B. Saunders Co. 1986; p. 1095.

3 *Cecil's Textbook of Medicine*, 18th edition, 1988; pg. 1514.

4 *Harrison's Principles of Internal Medicine*, 12th edition, 1991; p. 1295.

5 *Scientific American Medicine*, updated, chapter 15, section X, p. 9.

6 Barzel U.S. 'Estrogens in the prevention and treatment of postmenopausal osteoporosis:a review'. *Am J Med* 1988;85:847-850.

7 Felson D.R., Zhang Y., Hannan M.T., et al. 'The effect of postmenopausal estrogen therapy on bone density in elderly women'. *N Engl J Med* 1993; 329: 1141-1146.

8 Gambrell R.D. 'The menopause: benefits and risks of estrogen-progestogen replacement therapy'. *Fertil Steril* 1983;37:457-474.

9 Lee J.R. 'Osteoporosis reversal: the role of progesterone'. *Intern Clin Nutr Rev* 1990;10:384-391.

2. What is progesterone?

Reference texts used:

Goodman & Gilman, *The Pharmacological Basis of Therapeutics*, 8th edition, 1990; Chapter 58.

Textbook of Clinical Chemistry, editor Norbert W. Tietz, PhD, W.B. Saunders Co. 1986; pp. 1085-1171.

Will's Biochemical Basis of Medicine, second edition, Wright, 1989; Chapter 17.

3. What are progestins?

1 Ottoson U.B., Johansson B.G., von Schoultz B. 'Subfractions of high-density lipoprotein cholesterol during estrogen replacement therapy: a comparison between progestogens and natural progesterone'. *Am J. Obstet Gynecol* 1985; 151:746-750.

2   Hargrove J.T., Maxson W.S., Wentz A.C., Burnett L.S. 'Menopausal hormone replacement therapy with continuous daily oral micronized estradiol and progesterone'. *OB&Gyn* 1989; 71:606-612.

3   Stevenson J.C., Ganger K.F., et al. 'Effects of transdermal versus oral hormone replacement therapy on bone density in spine and proximal femur in postmenopausal women'. *Lancet* 1990; 336:265-269.

4   Whitehead M.I., Fraser D., Schenkel L., Crook D., Stevenson J.C. 'Transdermal administration of oestrogen/progestagen hormone replacement therapy'. *Lancet* 1990; 335:310-312.

5   Crane M.G., Harris J.J. 'Effects of gonadal hormones on plasma renin activity and aldosterone excretion rate'. In: Salhanick H.A.,Kipnis D.M., Vande Weile R.L., eds: *Metabolic effects of gonadal hormones and contraceptive steroids*. Plenum Press, NY, 1969; 446-463, and Discussion, p. 736.

6   Crane Mg, Harris J.J., Winsor W. III. 'Hypertension, oral contraceptive agents, and conjugated estrogens'. *Ann Int Med* 1971; 74:13-21.

7   Landau R.L., Lugibihl K. 'The catabolic and natriuretic effects of progesterone in man'. *Recent Progr. Horm. Res.* 1961; 17:249-281.

8   Edgren R.A. *Progestagens.* Reprinted from *Clinical Use of Sex Steroids*, Yearbook Medical Publishers, Inc., 1980.

9   *Scientific American Medicine*, updated 1992, chapter 15, section X, p. 9.

10 Gambrell R.D. 'The menopause: benefits & risks of estrogen-progestogen replace-ment therapy'. *Medical Times* 1989 Sept; 35-43.

11 Bergkvist L., Adami H.-O., Persson I., Hoover R., Schairer C. 'The risk of breast cancer after estrogen and estrogen-progestin replacement'. *N Engl J Med* 1989; 321:293-297

4. The dance of the steroids

1   Gaby Alan R. *Preventing and Reversing Osteoporosis*, Prima Publishing, 1994.

5. Progesterone and the menstrual cycle

1   Prior J.C., Vigna Y.M. 'Spinal bone loss and ovulatory disturbances'. *N Engl J Med* 1990; 223:1221-1227.

2   Prior J.C., Vigna Y.M., Alojado N. 'Progesterone and the prevention of osteoporosis'. *Canadian J of Ob/Gyn & Women Health Care* 1991; 3:178-184.

3   Prior JC. 'Progesterone as a bone-trophic hormone'. *Endocrine Reviews*

1990; 11:386-398.

6. Progesterone and pregnancy

1   Campbell B.C., Ellison B.T. 'Menstrual variation in salivary testosterone among regularly cycling women'. *Horm Res* (Switzerland) 1992; 37(4-5): 132-6. ISSN 0301-0163.

7. Progesterone and menopause

1   te Velde E.R. (letter) 'Disappearing ovarian follicles and reproductive aging'. *Lancet* 1993; 341: 1125.

2   Leridon H. *Human fertility: the basic components.* Chicago: University of Chicago Press, 1977:202.

3   Van Noord-Zaadstra BM, Looman CWN, Alsback H, et al. 'Delaying childbearing: effect of age on fecundity and outcome of pregnancy'. *BMJ* 1991; 302: 1361-1365.

8. A word about oestrogen

1   Sheehy G. *The Silent Passage,* Pocket Books 1991; p. 24.

2   Raloff J. 'EcoCancers'. *Science News* 3 July 1993; 144:10-13.

3   Reported in article, 'Sperm-count drop tied to pollution rise', *Medical Tribune,* 26 March 1992.

4   Documenta Geigy, *Scientific Tables* sixth edition; p. 493.

5   Lennon H.M., Wotiz H.H., Parsons L., Mozden P.J. 'Reduced estriol excretion in patients with breast cancer prior to endocrine therapy'. *JAMA* 1966; 196:112-120.

6   Raz R., Stamm W.E. 'A controlled trial of intravaginal estriol in post-menopausal women with recurrent urinary tract infections'. *N Engl J Med* 1993; 329: 753-756.

7   Felson D.T., Zhang Y., Hannan M.T., Kiel D.P., Wilson P.W.F., Anderson J.J. 'The effect of postmenopausal estrogen therapy on bone density in elderly women'. *N Engl J Med* 1993; 329:1141-1146.

8   Cummings S. R. et al. 'Endogenous hormones and the risk of hip and vertebral fractures among older women'. *N Eng J Med,* 10 September 1998, 339:733-738.

9   Prior J. C. 'Perimenopause: the complex endocrinology of the menopausal transition'. *Endocrine Reviews* 1998; 19 (4):397-426.

10 Personal correspondence with the author.

11 Hulley S. et al. 'Randomized trial of estrogen plus progestin for secondary prevention of coronary heart disease in postmenopausal women'. *JAMA*, 19 August 1998; 280:605-613.

9. Progesterone and pelvic disorders

1 See reference 6 above, Chapter 8.

10. Progesterone and PMS

1 Reported in article, 'Progesterone: Safe Antidote for PMS', in *McCall's*, October 1990, pp. 152-156.

2 This chapter relies on my own clinical experience in using natural progesterone for patients with PMS.

11. Progesterone and osteoporosis

1 Albright F., Smith P.H., Richardson A.M. 'Postmenopausal osteoporosis: its clinical features'. *JAMA* 1941; 116:2465-2474.

2 Aitken M., Hart D.M., Lindsay R. 'Oestrogen replacement therapy for prevention of osteoporosis after oopherectomy'. *Br Med J* 1973; 3:515-518.

3 Lindsay R., Hart D.M., Forrest C., Baird C. 'Prevention of spinal osteoporosis in oophorectomized women'. *Lancet* 1980; II:1151-1154.

4 Gordon G.S., Picchi J., Root B.S. 'Antifracture efficacy of long-term estrogens for osteoporosis'. *Trans Assoc Am Physicians* 1973; 86:326-332.

5 Hammond C.B., Jelvsek F.R., Lee K.L., Creasman W.T., Parker R.T. 'Effects of long-term estrogen replacement therapy. I. Metabolic effects'. *Am J Ob-Gyn* 1979; 133:525-536.

6 Hutchinson T.A., Polansky S.M., Feinstein A.R. 'Postmenopausal oestrogens protect against fractures of hip and distal radius: a case control study'. *Lancet* 1979; II: 705-709.

7 Weiss N.S., Ure C.L., Ballard J.H., Williams A.R., Daling J.R. 'Decreased risk of fracture of hip and lower forearm with postmenopausal use of estrogen'. *N Engl J Med* 1980; 303:1195-1198.

8 Ettinger B., Genant H.K., Cann C.E. 'Long-term estrogen replacement therapy prevents bone loss and fractures'. *Ann Intern Med* 1985; 102:319-324.

9 Barzel U.S. 'Estrogens in the prevention and treatment of postmenopausal osteo-porosis: a review'. *Am J Med* 1988; 85:847-850.

10 Christiansen C., Christiansen M.S., Transbol I. 'Bone mass in post-menopausal women after withdrawal of oestrogen/gestagen replacement therapy'. *Lancet* 1981 Feb 28; 459-461.

11 Prior J.C., Vigna V.M. 'Spinal bone loss and ovulatory disturbances'. *N Engl J Med* 1990; 323:1221-1227.

12 Rudy D.R. 'Hormone replacement therapy'. *Postgraduate Medicine* 1990 Dec; 157-164.

13 Dargent-Molina P., Favier F., Grandjean H., Baudoin C., Schott A.M., Hausherr E., Meunier P.J., Bréart G., for the EPIDOS Group. 'Fall-related factors and risk of hip fracture: the EPIDOS prospective study'. *The Lancet* 1996; 348: 145-149.

14 Cummings S.R., Mevitt M.C., Browner W.S. et al for the Study of Osteoporotic Fractures Research Group. 'Risk factors for hip fracture in white women'. *N Engl J Med* 1995; 332: 767-773.

15 Felson D.T., Zhang Y., Hannan M.T., Kiel D.P., Wilson P.W.F., Anderson J.J. 'The effect of postmenopausal estrogen therapy on bone density in elderly women'. *N Engl J Med* 1993; 329:1141-1146.

16 Manolagas S.C., Jilka R.L., Hangoc G., et al. 'Increased osteoclast development after estrogen loss: mediation by interleukin-6'. *Science* 1992; 257:88-91.

17 Prior J.C. 'Progesterone as a bone-trophic hormone'. *Endocrine Reviews* 1990; 11: 386-398.

18 Prior J.C., Vigna Y.M., Burgess R. 'Medroxyprogesterone acetate increases trabecular bone density in women with menstrual disorder'. Presented at the annual meeting of the Endocrine Society, June 11, 1987, Indianapolis.

19 Munk-Jensen N., Nielsen S.P., Obel E.B., Eriksen P.B. 'Reversal of post-menopausal vertebral bone loss by oestrogen and progestagen: a double-blind placebo-controlled study'. *Br Med J* 1988; 296:1150-1152.

20 Johansen J.S., Jensen S.B., Riis B.J., et al. 'Bone formation is stimulated by combined estrogen, progestagen'. *Metabolism* 1990; 39:1122-1126.

21 Cundy T., Evans M., Roberts H., et al. 'Bone density in women receiving a depot medroxyprogesterone acetate for contraception'. *Br Med J 1991*; 303:13-16.

22 Lee J.R. 'Osteoporosis reversal: the role of progesterone'. *Intern Clin Nutr Rev* 1990; 10:384-391.

23 Lee J.R. 'Osteoporosis reversal with transdermal progesterone' (letter).

Lancet 1990; 336:1327

24 Lee J.R. 'Is natural progesterone the missing link in osteoporosis prevention and treatment?' *Medical Hypotheses* 1991; 35:316-318.

25 *Will's Biochemical Basis of Medicine* 1989, chapter 22, p. 258.

26 Lees B., Molleson T., Arnett T.R., Stevenson J.C. 'Differences in proximal femur density over two centuries'. *Lancet* 1993; 341:673-675.

27 Coats C. 'Negative effects of a high-protein diet'. *Family Practice Recertification* 1990; 12:80-88.

28 Riggs B.L., Hodgson S.F., O'Fallon W.M., Chao E.Y.S., et al. 'Effect of fluoride treatment on the fracture rate in postmenopausal women with osteoporosis'. *N Engl J Med* 1990; 322:802-809.

29 Kleerekoper M.E., Peterson E., Phillips E., Nelson D., et al. 'Continuous sodium fluoride therapy does not reduce vertebral fracture rate in postmenopausal osteoporosis'. [abstract] *J Bone & Miner Res* 1989; Res. 4 (Suppl. 1):S376.

30 Hedlund L.R., Gallagher J.C. 'Increased incidence of hip fracture in osteoporotic women treated with sodium fluoride'. *J Bone & Miner Res* 1989; 4:223-225.

31 Sowers M.F.R., Clark M.K., Jannausch M.L., Wallace R.B. 'A prospective study of bone mineral content and fracture in communities with differential fluoride exposure'. *Am J Epidemiol* 1991; 134:649-660.

32 Jacobsen S.J., Goldberg J., Miles T.P., Brody J.A., et al. 'Regional variation in the incidence of hip fractures; US white women aged 65 years and older'. *JAMA* 1990; 264:500-502.

33 Cooper C., Wickham C.A.C., Barker D.J.R., Jacobsen S.J. 'Water fluoridation and hip fracture'. (Letter) *JAMA* 1991; 266:513-514.

34 Danielson C., Lyon J.L., Egger M., Goodenough G.K. 'Hip fractures and fluoridation in Utah's elderly population'. *JAMA* 1992; 268:746-747.

12. Progesterone and Cancer

1 Bergkvist L., Adami H.-O., Persson I., Hoover R., Schairer C. 'The risk of breast cancer after estrogen and estrogen-progestin replacement'. *N Engl J Med* 1989; 321:293-297.

2 Henderson B.E., Ross R.K., Pike M.C., Casagrande J.T. 'Endogenous hormones as a major factor in human cancer'. *Cancer Res* 1982; 42:3232-3239.

3 Hoover R., Gray L.A. Sr, Cole P., MacMahon B. 'Menopausal estrogens

and breast cancer'. *N Engl J Med* 1976; 295:401-405.

4   Hiatt R.A., Bawol R., Friedman G.D., Hoover R. 'Exogenous estrogen and breast cancer after bilateral oophorectomy'. *Cancer* 1984; 54:139-144.

5   La Vecchia C., Decarli A., Parazzini F., Gentile A., Liberati C., Franceschi S. 'Non-contraceptive oestrogens and the risk of breast cancer in women'. *Int J Cancer* 1986; 38:853-858.

6   Cowan L.D., Gordis L., Tonascia J.A., Jones G.S. 'Breast cancer incidence in women with a history of progesterone deficiency'. *Am J Epidemiology* 1981; 114:209-217.

7   A report by Ruby Senie, PhD, of the Centres for Disease Control, at the annual science writers seminar sponsored by the American Cancer Society. Reported by the February 5, 1992, issue of *HEALTH* and by the May 7, 1992, issue of *Medical Tribune*.

8   Janet Raloff. 'EcoCancers: do environmental factors underlie a breast cancer epidemic?' *Science News* 3 July 1993; 144:10-13.

9   Lemon H.M., Wotiz H.H., Parsons L., Mozden P.J. 'Reduced estriol excretion in patients with breast cancer prior to endocrine therapy'. *JAMA* 1966; 196:112-120.

10 Cowan L.D., Gordis L., Tonascia J.A., Jones G.S. 'Breast cancer incidence in women with a history of progesterone deficiency'. *Am J Epidemiology* 1981; 114: 209-217.

11 Personal correspondence with the author.

12 Hrushesky W.J.M. 'Breast cancer, timing of surgery, and the menstrual cycle: call for prospective trial'. *J Women's Health* 1996; 5: 555-566.

13 Mohr P.E., Wang D.Y.,Gregory W.M., Richards M.A., Fentiman I.S. 'Serum progesterone and prognosis in operable breast cancer'. *British J Cancer* 1996; 73: 1552-1555.

14 Formby B. and Wiley T.S. 'Progesterone inhibits growth and induces apoptosis in breast cancer cells: Inverse effect on expression of p53 and Bcl-2'. Sansum Medical Research Foundation, Santa Barbara, California. Awaiting publication.

15 Cavalieri E.L., Stack D.E., Devanesan P.D., Todorovic R. et al. 'Molecular origin of cancer: Catechol estrogen-3,4-quinones as endogenous tumor initiators'. *Proc Natl Acad Sci* 997; 94: 10937-10942.

16 Chang K.-J., Lee T.T.Y., Linares-Cruz G., Fournier S., de Lignieres B. 'Influences of percutaneous administration of estradiol and progesterone on human breast epithelial cell cycle in vivo. *Fertility and Sterility*

1995; 63:785-791.

17 Rodriques C., Calle E.E., Loates R.J. et al. 'Estrogen replacement therapy and fatal ovarian cancer'. *American J Epidemiology* 141: 828-834, 1995

18 Cavalieri E.L., Stack D.E., Devanesan P.D. et al. 'Molecular origin of cancer: Catechol estrogen-3,4-quinones as endogenous tumor indicators'. *Proc Natl Acad Sci* 94: 10937-10942, 1997.

13. Women's heart disease and hormones

1   Miyagawa K., Rosch J., Stancyk F. & Hersmeyer K. 'Medroxyprogesterone interferes with ovarian protection against coronary vasospasm'. *Nature Medicine* 1997; 3:324-327.

2   Williams J.K., Honore E.K., Washburn S.A. & Clarkson T.B. 'Effects of hormone replacement therapy on reactivity of atherosclerotic coronary arteries in cynomolgus monkeys'. *J Am Coll Cardiology* 1994; 24:1757-1761.

3   'Hormone Therapy: Issues of the Heart'. *Science News*, 8 March 1997, vol 151, page 140.

14. Prostate problems and hormones

15. How to use natural progesterone

My references here are my own experience in using natural progesterone since 1982.

Afterword

1   Ellison P.T., Painter-Brick C., Lipson S.F., O'Rourke M.T. 'The ecological context of human ovarian function'. *Hum Reprod Dec* 1993;8(12):2248-58

2   Ellison P.T. 'Measurments of salivary progesterone'. *Ann NY Acad Sci* Sept 20, 1993; 694:161-76.

3   Ellison P.T., Lipson S.F., O'Rourke M.T., et al. 'Population variation in ovarian function' (letter). *Lancet* Aug 14, 1993;342:433-4.

4   Campbell B.C., Ellison P.T. 'Menstrual variation in salivary testosterone among regularly cycling women'. *Horm Res* (Switzerland) 1992;37:(4-5):132-6.

5   PEPI Trial writing group. 'Effect of estrogen or estrogen/progestin reminens on heart disease risk fctors in postmenopausal women'. *JAMA* Jan

18, 1995;273:199-208.

6   Prior J.C. 'Progesterone and its role in bone remodeling'. Chapter 3 of *Sex Steroids and Bone*, Springer-Verlag, 1994.

7   Cummings S.R., Nevitt M.C., Browner W.S., et al. 'Risk factors for hip fracture in white women'. *New Eng J Med* March 23, 1995;332:767-73.

Further information

Suggested reading

What Your Doctor May Not Tell You About Menopause, Dr John Lee and Virginia Hopkins, Warner Books, 1996.

Premenopause: What Your Doctor May Not Tell You, Dr John Lee, Dr Jesse Hanley and Virginia Hopkins, Warner Books, 1999.

Natural Progesterone, AnnA Rushton and Dr Shirley A. Bond, Thorsons, 1999.

My Body, My Health: The concerned woman's guide to gynecology, Felicia Stewart MD, Felicia Guest, Gary Stewart MD, and Robert Hatcher MD. John Wiley & Sons, 1979.

What's Wrong with My Hormones? Gillian Ford. Desmond Ford Publications, 7955 Bullard Drive, Newcastle, CA 95658, 1992.

Super Nutrition for Menopause, by Ann Louise Gittleman. Pocket Books, 1993.

Hormone Replacement Therapy: Yes or No? Betty Kamen. Nutrition Encounter, Inc., P.O. Box 5847, Novato, CA 94948, 1993.

Preventing and Reversing Osteoporosis, Alan R. Gaby MD. Prima Publishing, P.O. Box 1260BK, Rocklin, CA 95677, 1993.

Women's Bodies, Women's Wisdom, Christiane Northrup MD. Bantam Books.

Breezing Through the Change, Ellen Brown & Lynne Walker. Frog, Ltd., P.O. Box 12327, Berkeley, CA.

A Passage to Power: Natural Menopause Revolution, Leslie Kenton. Ebury Press, London.

Balancing Hormones Naturally, Kate Neil. ION Press, 13 Blades Court, Deodar Road, London SW15 2NU.

The John R. Lee MD Medical Letter, an informative newsletter on topics relating to progesterone and health published by Dr Lee in the US, is available on subscription from the NPIS (see below).

Information and advice

The following information has been compiled by the publisher for the
UK edition of this book. All was believed accurate at the time of
publication, but readers should confirm the facts for themselves before
placing orders. The publisher cannot be held responsible for errors.

The Natural Progesterone Information Service (NPIS), PO Box 24, Buxton
SK17 9FB (www.npis.info) offers a comprehensive information pack for
women, including a detailed fact sheet, answers to common questions, a list
of doctors who prescribe progesterone, and interesting articles, plus a list of
books, audio and video tapes available on this subject. NPIS also supply a
doctor's information pack. Please send a 1st class stamp for full information.

Woman to Woman conducts hormonal seminars, publishes *Healthy News for
Women* and sells health books. For a sample newsletter and product list, send
an SAE to Woman to Woman, PO Box 2252, Hove, BN3 6BU.

The **Well Woman's International Network (WWIN)** is a subscriber organi-
sation that publishes a newsletter acting as a forum for PMS, pre- and
post-menopause and osteoporosis sufferers. www.nhmworldwide.co.uk

The Natural Health Ministry, Well Woman Nutrition Centre, Gort Loskey,
Donegal, Co Donegal, Eire. www.nhmworldwide.co.uk From the UK tel 0701
070 3124 (24 hrs), fax 0701 070 3456. (From outside the UK dial +44 701…).
The Natural Health Ministry supplies Pro-Gest Cream and Oil and Es-Gen
Cream by mail order to individuals anywhere in the world, including the UK,
without a prescription.

Wellsprings Serenity is a pure, bio-identical natural progesterone cream
formulated to a recipe approved by Dr John Lee since 1995. Wellsprings offers
global delivery and orders can be placed on their website or by calling their
contact centre. www.serenityprogesterone.com www.progesterone.co.uk
Tel +44 (0)1481 233370

Index

E1, *see* oestrone
E2, *see* oestradiol
E3, *see* oestriol
Ellison, Dr Peter, 34, 127-8
endocrine system, 90
endometriosis, 56, 59-61
enzymes, 15, 25, 28, 78, 80, 82
ethinyloestradiol, hazards of, 49,
    50, 52, 54, 114
evolution, 5

fat, body, 49
fatigue, 27, 40, 42, 64-5, 103
fatty acids, 10, 43, 93, 123
FDA, 2, 110
feeling cold, 42
fibrocystic breasts, 3, 9, 14, 41, 44,
    50, 55, 62, 68, 118, 120-1
fibroids, *see* uterine fibroid tumours
folic acid, 105, 123
Fosamax, 71, 72, 74
FSH, 15, 30-2, 42-3, 45, 51, 58, 59,
    65, 122-3

Gaby, Dr. Alan, 27
genes, 5, 6, 38, 64, 67, 87-8, 91, 92-
    3, 108
gestagens, 7, 17, 47
GnRH, *see* gonadotropin-releasing
    hormone
gonadotropin-releasing hormone,
    30, 32
gonadotropins, 21, 30-1, 42, 64

hair, body, 40, 42; facial, 26, 41, 42;
    scalp, 26; pubic, 29
Hargrove, Dr. Joel T., 19, 66, 111
headaches, 50, 51, 52, 64, 65
heart disease, 53-4, 84, 98, 102-5
herbal remedies, 54, 122, 144
hot flushes, 22, 39, 40, 42, 45, 51,
    52, 53, 68, 71, 118
Hrushesky, William J.M., 91-2
hypertension, 3, 9, 12, 20-1, 52, 119
hyperthyroidism and osteoporosis,
    86, 117

hypothalamus, 28, 30-3, 44
hypothyroidism, 3, 37, 42, 65, 117

IgA, 57
immune system, 27, 57, 92, 117
interleukin, 75, 79, 92
iron, 105

LH (luteinizing hormone), 15, 30-2,
    42-5, 51, 58-9, 65, 122-3
libido, 2, 3, 12-14, 39, 44, 45, 50,
    62, 64-5, 97-8
limbic brain, 28, 30, 32, 42
liver, 6, 8, 11, 12, 14, 16, 19, 25, 26,
    33, 48, 52, 66, 68, 82, 96, 111,
    114
luteal phase of menstrual cycle, 30,
    36, 71, 91

magnesium, 20, 43, 58, 67, 78-80,
    82, 86, 104, 118, 122, 123
Manolagas et al, 75
memory, 27
menopause, 9-46, *passim*
menstrual cycle, 29-33, *passim*
metabolic acidosis, 85
miscarriage, 34-6
mistletoe, 1-2
mittelschmerz, 56, 58-9
mood swings, 39, 42, 44

obesity, 27, 105, 119
oestradiol, 19, 22, 26, 29, 47-55, 89-
    90, 92-8, 100-1, 103-4, 108, 109,
    114, 118, 145
oestriol, 26, 46, 48, 49, 54-5, 57, 58,
    59, 89-90, 93, 96, 97, 101, 109,
    118, 123, 145
oestrogen, 47-55, 88-90, *passim*;
    dominance, 44-5, 50; effects of,
    passim; dosage 51-5; unopposed,
    9, 12, 14, 22, 32, 50, 62, 68, 87,
    89, 92, 96, 97, 100, 101, 108,
    116
oestrone, 26, 46, 48, 49, 52, 54-5,
    58, 89-90, 93, 96-7, 101, 104,